Orthopedic Advisor

So You Have Osteoporosis… Now What?

Orthopedic Advisor

So You Have Osteoporosis… Now What?

Andrew J. Cozadd, PA-C
Orthopedic Surgery
Minneapolis, Minnesota

Orthopedic Advisor

So You Have Osteoporosis... Now What?

About the Author

Andrew Cozadd is an orthopedic PA with a passion for education and bone health. In addition to managing the full spectrum of orthopedic conditions, he pioneered an osteoporosis program to better serve the needs of the community. Osteoporosis combines his passion for fracture management and all of the complex medical pathophysiology that sparked his initial interest in medicine. His first text entitled **Osteoporosis: The Clinician's Guide to Diagnosis and Management** has been a valued resource for medical providers managing osteoporosis. His most recent text, **So You Have Osteoporosis... Now What?** was written to entertain, educate, and empower patients to make well informed decisions regarding their bone health based on the most up-to-date information from the medical community. Please do not hesitate to contact Andrew Cozadd at orthopedic.advisor@gmail.com with questions, comments, or personal triumphs! Together, we can manage osteoporosis!

Table of Contents

Preface

When broken down into its most basic elements, osteoporosis is a rather simple concept to grasp. Despite this simplicity, few would argue against the fact that osteoporosis is a rather complex condition to fully understand. Rarely does a single visit to your medical provider's office provide all of the details necessary to feel confident in knowing not just the "what," but the "how" and the "why" of osteoporosis care. I am often asked by my patients what text I would recommend for further reading on osteoporosis—a fair question that I put great effort into researching. After searching high and low for what I believed the be the perfect text—one that was objective and filled with research supported facts and free of sensationalized claims, one that was thorough enough to answer all of the pertinent questions without being written at a level only those with Ph. D's could grasp, I was disappointed in the available options. The task of writing such a text is one that I did not take lightly. My goal in writing this text was to provide the most up to date information regarding the questions that you need to know about osteoporosis. After reading this text, you will be armed with all of the necessary information to make well informed and scientifically supported decisions regarding your osteoporosis care.

1 | Let's Start with the Basics

What is osteoporosis?

The first question that I am often asked by patients is, "What exactly is osteoporosis?" The answer to this question lies in the origin of the word. When broken down into its components, "osteo-" refers to bone, and "-porosis" refers to the condition of being porous or full of holes. Quite literally, osteoporosis means porous bone – a disease in which the bones that make up the skeletal system become weak and brittle. Those suffering from this disease are more likely experience a broken bone, which is commonly referred to as a fracture in the medical community. People with osteoporosis have bones that are made up of all of the right building blocks; there simply is a reduced amount of bone present.[1]

What are my chances of developing osteoporosis?

Osteoporosis is a common disease that has become increasingly more prevalent as medical advances have allowed for longer life expectancies. It is estimated that over 10 million people in the United States, and over 200 million people worldwide currently suffer from this disease.[2,1] While many of these people are completely unaware that they have osteoporosis and may never experience a fracture, others are not so fortunate. Weakened bones from osteoporosis cause fractures in 30-40% of postmenopausal women and 15-30% of men over 50 years old.[3,4] To put it into perspective, osteoporosis related fractures are more common than heart attacks, stroke, and new cases of breast cancer combined! Each year over 1.5 million people in the United States and 8.9 million people worldwide with osteoporosis will fracture – which means that osteoporosis causes a fracture every 3 seconds![2,5] After the first broken bone, the risk of sustaining a second within the next year increases 86%.[6] To make matters worse, the rate of fractures caused by osteoporosis is only increasing... By 2050, the worldwide incidence of hip fracture is projected to increase by 310% and 240% in men and women, respectively.[7] While there is no cure for osteoporosis, all hope is not lost! There are treatments available to improve bone strength and decrease the risk of broken bones! It should feel empowering to know that you can take control of your bone health!

What is a fragility fracture?

Osteoporosis is generally a silent disease – meaning that those with osteoporosis do not have any physical symptoms. Patients do not walk into the office saying that their osteoporosis is flaring up. As you can imagine, this makes the diagnosis of osteoporosis tricky! The goal of medical providers is to identify patients with osteoporosis through routine screenings before a fracture happens. However, it is not uncommon for a fracture to be our first clue of underlying osteoporosis, particularly in the orthopedic world.

Not all broken bones are concerning for osteoporosis, but certain types of broken bones known as "fragility fractures" are suspicious for underlying osteoporosis. A **fragility fracture** is a broken bone that occurs from a physiologic stress that we would not expect to lead to fracture in a person with healthy, strong bones. Fragility fractures typically involve a fall from a standing height leading to a fracture in one of the following bones, which happen to be the most vulnerable bones in those with osteoporosis.

- **SHOULDER** (proximal humerus fracture)
- **WRIST** (distal radius fracture)
- **HIP** (femoral neck or intertrochanteric femur fractures)
- **PELVIS** (pubic rami or sacral fractures)
- **SPINE** (vertebral compression fracture)

The concept of a fragility fracture is often confusing for patients. When they recall how they broke a bone, most will emphasize how hard the ground was, or how much force was involved during the fall. There is occasionally even an element of denial that their injury should be classified as a fragility fracture. I get it! By no means is your medical provider minimizing your injury – you broke a bone and last I checked, that is a painful injury! Let's take a look at a couple scenarios to better illustrate what qualifies as a fragility fracture.

Mary is a 45 year old female who is driving down the highway when she crashes into the median at high speeds. As a result, she sustains a shoulder and hip fracture. She is rushed to the hospital for medical attention. Due to the high energy nature of this crash, these fractures are not concerning for osteoporosis. Likewise, Mark is a 60 year old male who did not listen to his wife and decided to clean out the gutters on his own instead of hiring a company to do so. While standing on the top step of his ladder he falls, breaking his right wrist. Again, this would not be considered a fragility fracture because Mark fell from a significant height.

Now let's look at Tim, a 65 year old male who is walking down his icy concrete driveway to check the mail. He falls and lands hard on his right side. During the fall, he sustains a hip fracture. Since he fell from a standing height and broke his hip, this is classified as a fragility fracture and requires further evaluation for osteoporosis.

How does osteoporosis develop?

To understand how osteoporosis develops, we must first take an in-depth look at the nuts and bolts of the human skeleton. When you think of bone, what comes to mind? Do you picture a hard, inanimate object made up of calcium to help support your body? That is the typical answer. While this view is not entirely wrong, and bones do store 99% of the body's calcium reserves, it is much too simplified. Below I will discuss the most important components of bone and how they relate to osteoporosis.

- If you were to saw a bone in half and look at it with the naked eye, you would see that bones have a dense outer shell known as **cortical** bone, and a less dense, inner lattice-like structure known as **trabecular** or **cancellous** bone.

- If you look at this same bone under a microscope, two types of cells with very important functions exist: **osteoblasts** and **osteoclasts**. More on these in just a second!

- Bone is an active organ system that undergoes a constant process of **remodeling** – meaning old and damaged bone is replaced with new and healthy bone. This process occurs throughout our entire lives and is necessary to repair the daily damage that our bones endure!

- **Osteoclast** cells are the bone recyclers. They are responsible for breaking down old and damaged bone in a process called **bone resorption.**

- **Osteoblast** cells are the bone builders. They are responsible for creating new and healthy bone in a process called **bone ossification.**

The bone building osteoblasts and bone recycling osteoclasts communicate with one another to ensure that the rate of bone recycling and the rate of new bone being created are equal and well-coordinated. The osteoblasts are the generals who lead the way – these cells release a chemical message called **RANKL** which acts as an "ON" signal for the osteoclast cells to begin breaking down old bone. Osteoblasts also release another chemical message called **OPG** which acts as an "OFF" signal for osteoclasts to stop breaking down old bone. This allows the osteoblasts to fill in the region with new, healthy bone.[8] **An imbalance between the rate of old bone being broken down and new bone being created can lead to a loss of bone density over time and ultimately, osteoporosis.**

The density of our bones fluctuates in a relatively predictable manner throughout our lives. Bones increase in strength throughout adolescence, particularly during our early teenage years, and reach peak density by the time we reach 30 years old.[9] At this point, our bones are strong and require a significant amount of force to break. Beyond 30 years old, our bone density begins to slowly decline due to normal aging and those bone reserves that were built during adolescence are put to the test. There are a number of factors which can impair our ability to build strong bones during adolescence, including genetics, ethnicity, poor calcium and vitamin D intake, underlying medical conditions and use of certain medications. If our peak bone density is insufficient due to any of these reasons, then the completely normal age-related bone loss could lead to our bones becoming brittle and more prone to fracturing in later life. To illustrate this point, let's consider the following analogy.

Picture your bone reserves as a piggy bank. If you continually add to your piggy bank throughout your childhood years, you might save up $100 worth of "stored bone." However, if you forget to take the necessary steps to add to your piggy bank, you might only save up $50 worth of "stored bone." Now we hit 30 years of age and no more money can be added! We start pulling from the piggy bank at a rate of $2 per year. For the person that saved $100 worth of bone, it will take 50 years before they run out of bone reserves. This would lead to the development of osteoporosis at age 80. For the person that only saved up $50 worth of bone, they would only have 25 years until osteoporosis develops at age 55!

Certain events can dramatically accelerate the speed at which we lose bone density– the most common of which is menopause in women. When women enter menopause, there is a decrease in the amount of the hormone estrogen produced by the body. Estrogen has a number of important functions in maintaining bone health. Estrogen increases the activity of the osteoblast "bone builder" cells and decreases the activity of the osteoclast "bone recycler" cells.[10] When estrogen is lost, instead of an even rate of bone building and recycling, the pendulum swings to favor bone recycling, which exceeds the rate at which new bone can be formed. Starting 2-3 years before menopause and ending 3-4 years after, women lose an average of 10.5% of their spine bone density, and 5.3% of the density in their hips.[11] This abrupt loss of bone density, combined with the normal progressive age related bone loss makes women more susceptible to developing osteoporosis at a younger age compared to men. Men are not completely out of the woods when it comes to osteoporosis – but they generally develop osteoporosis 10 years later than women.

Aside from menopause, other factors can influence the rate in which bone is lost over time, as well as how likely a person is to sustain a fragility fracture. Let us begin with the risk factors that you have no control over – I will refer to these as **nonmodifiable risk factors**.[12]

- **GENETICS.** You can thank your parents for this one. Family history of osteoporosis and fragility fractures increases your risk of developing osteoporosis.

- **ETHNICITY.** Osteoporosis is more common in Caucasian and Asian populations.

- **AGE.** As we discussed above, we will all experience a predictable loss of bone density after we reach 30 years of age. The older we become, the greater the risk of osteoporosis and fractures.

- **GENDER.** Women experience menopause, and therefore have a greater risk of developing osteoporosis at a younger age compared to men.

- **PREVIOUS FRACTURE.** There is no changing the fact that you had a prior fracture, and when it comes to broken bones, one fracture can start a snowball effect and increase your odds of another.

- **RHEUMATOID ARTHRITIS.** This is a form of arthritis in which the body's immune system attacks the joints and other body tissues. This can cause significant inflammation within the body, which can lead to bone breakdown. People with rheumatoid arthritis have been shown to have an increased risk of developing osteoporosis.

There is certainly a lot that we cannot control. If you read the list above and thought to yourself "Here we go! I have multiple risk factors for osteoporosis that I can't even control!" you are not alone. But all hope is not lost! You may find it empowering to know that there are **modifiable risk factors** – or those that you have complete control over![12]

- **ALCOHOL.** Consuming more than two alcoholic beverages daily leads to a 40% increased risk of fragility fracture.[13]

- **SMOKING.** Smoking one pack of cigarettes daily in adult life leads to a 5-10% loss of bone density and increased risk of fracture.[14,15]

- **LOW BODY MASS INDEX (BMI).** The body mass index is a measure of how much you weigh and your height. Low weight for your height, as indicated by a BMI below 20, increases your risk of sustaining a fracture. Interestingly, those who are overweight have a decreased risk of developing osteoporosis… but don't take this as advice to be overweight! There are far healthier ways to improve your bone health!

- **NUTRITION.** People who are deficient in calcium (a necessary building block for strong bones) and vitamin D (which helps our body absorb calcium from the foods we eat) are at increased risk for developing osteoporosis.

- **INSUFFICIENT EXERCISE.** Weight bearing exercise including walking, resistance exercises, and aerobic training may improve bone density, muscular strength, and decrease the risk of falls.

- **FREQUENT FALLS.** If you are simply clumsy, be more mindful of your surroundings. If you have a medical condition which predisposes you to falls, then physical therapy, bracing, and other options may reduce this risk and should be considered.

How is osteoporosis classified?

Osteoporosis can be classified in two ways – by the type of osteoporosis that the patient has and by the severity of the disease.[16] In 1986, Riggs and Melton developed the following classification of osteoporosis which is still used today.

- **TYPE I PRIMARY OSTEOPOROSIS** is commonly known as postmenopausal osteoporosis. It affects women following the onset of menopause and is caused by the sudden loss of the hormone estrogen. This leads to a period of rapid bone loss. Women become most susceptible to fractures in bones that have a greater proportion of trabecular bone compared to cortical bone, including the spine and wrist.

- **TYPE II PRIMARY OSTEOPOROSIS** is commonly known as senile osteoporosis. It affects both men and women over age 70. There is a loss of both cortical and trabecular bone as a result of age-related bone loss. People are more susceptible to all types of fragility fractures with this form of osteoporosis.

- **SECONDARY OSTEOPOROSIS** is osteoporosis that develops due to an underlying medical condition or use of a medication known to weaken our bones. Secondary osteoporosis can affect men and women of all ages. It has been reported that up to 75% of men and 30-50% of women have a secondary cause for osteoporosis and that secondary osteoporosis accounts for up to 40% of all fragility fractures. [17-20]

While classifying osteoporosis based on type is a useful way to categorize people with the disease, the most common way to describe osteoporosis is based on how severely the bones are affected. The severity of osteoporosis is measured using a DXA bone density scan. This specialized x-ray of the hip, spine, or forearm provides useful information regarding the density of our bones. Results are reported in numeric T-scores, with more negative numbers representing weaker bones. This classification is commonly quoted by medical providers and patients alike. While it is a useful guide to roughly estimate fracture risk, many other factors must be considered when determining a patient's true risk of fracture, which will be discussed in later sections.

- **NORMAL BONE MINERAL DENSITY:** T-score +1.0 to -0.9
- **LOW BONE MINERAL DENSITY (OSTEOPENIA):** T-score -1.0 to -2.4
- **OSTEOPOROSIS:** T-score less than -2.5

Key Points

- Osteoporosis – literally meaning porous bone, is a common medical condition which results in decreased bone density (weakened bones) and increased risk of fracture.
- A fragility fracture involves a broken hip, wrist, spine, pelvis, or shoulder sustained during a fall from a standing height.
- Osteoporosis develops due to a variety of reasons, most of which are related to an imbalance between the rate that osteoclast cells break down old bone and osteoblast cells build new bone.
- People have the ability to increase bone density (increase their bone reserves) until they reach peak bone density at 30 years old – after which there is a normal, slow loss of bone density.
- Women experience a rapid loss of up to 10% or more of their bone density during menopause due to reduced estrogen – leading to the development of osteoporosis about 10 years earlier than men.
- Many modifiable and nonmodifiable risk factors exist which can speed up the rate in which bone is lost as we age.
- Osteoporosis is defined as a DXA measured T-score of -2.5 or less, but other factors need to be considered before determining your true risk of sustaining a fracture.

2 | Secondary Osteoporosis: the Bone Bandits

What is secondary osteoporosis?

Secondary osteoporosis is defined as low bone density caused by an underlying **medical condition** or use of a **medication** known to negatively impact bone health. This form of osteoporosis is not as rare as you might think! Researchers have been able to link secondary causes of osteoporosis to nearly 75% of men and 30-50% of women with osteoporosis.[21-23] Since the root cause is different than that seen in Type I and Type II osteoporosis, the treatment of secondary osteoporosis requires careful consideration. In some cases, proper treatment can cure the secondary cause of osteoporosis and improve your bone health! In others, no such cure is available, but measures can still be taken to maintain your bone density and decrease your risk of breaking bones.

Let's revisit the piggy bank analogy and take a look at how secondary causes of osteoporosis can affect our bone health. In the previous section we discussed a patient who was able to store $100 worth of bone. We know that after age 30, the slot on the top of our little piggy becomes sealed and we can no longer add new money. Instead, we spend $2 worth of bone each year due to normal age related bone loss. With secondary osteoporosis, the yearly fee increases. The cost varies because not all secondary causes affect our bones to the same degree. Some may only pull an additional $1 per year, whereas others may pull $10-20 per year! The patient with $100 in the piggy bank will continue to lose $2 yearly, but imagine if an additional $20 was pulled each year! Within a short period of time, this patient will develop osteoporosis if this goes unrecognized and untreated.

In this chapter I will provide a detailed review of medical conditions and medications which have been associated with osteoporosis. **Warning: this section is heavy on the medical terminology and is not for the faint of heart!** While I will make every effort to explain how these secondary causes of osteoporosis negatively impact your bone health, it is not important that you fully understand all of this information before moving on to the following chapters. In fact, understanding that secondary causes of osteoporosis exist and may impact your treatment options is all that you really need to know. Feel free to read any topics that you find interesting... and skip those that you don't!

If after browsing this section you recognize that you have been diagnosed with or experienced symptoms of any of these medical conditions, or if you are taking any of the medications listed, you should consider contacting your medical provider's office to discuss how your bone health may be impacted.

What medical conditions can cause secondary osteoporosis?

DIABETES MELLITUS (DM). There are two types of diabetes, both of which increase a patient's risk of developing osteoporosis and sustaining fragility fractures. **Type 1 diabetes** occurs when the body's immune system produces antibodies which attack the cells in the pancreas responsible for producing the hormone insulin – with the end result being a decrease in insulin production. Insulin allows our bodies to use sugar from the carbohydrates in our diet for energy. **Type 2 diabetes** occurs when organs stop responding appropriately to insulin. Both Type 1 and Type 2 diabetes lead to elevated blood sugar levels and symptoms such as increased thirst, hunger, frequent urination, and unexplained weight loss. Over time, diabetes can directly weaken bones and lead to nerve damage which effects balance and vision, making patients more likely to fall. People with Type 1 diabetes have a 12-fold greater risk of sustaining an osteoporosis related fracture compared to the general population, whereas those with Type 2 diabetes have a mildly increased risk of osteoporosis related fractures.[24] Excellent medical management of diabetes, including close monitoring of blood sugars, can decrease fracture risk.

HYPERTHYROIDISM. Hyperthyroidism occurs when the thyroid gland produces excessive amounts of thyroid hormone. Elevated levels of thyroid hormone are responsible for symptoms including a rapid heart rate (tachycardia), weight loss, restlessness, insomnia, protruding eyes (exophthalmos), and swelling in the lower legs. Hyperthyroidism has been shown to cause an increased rate of bone breakdown. Longstanding disease can increase the incidence of hip fractures 4-fold and spine fractures 5-fold compared to the general population.[25-26] Management of the underlying cause of hyperthyroidism, which may include medication and even surgery, can reverse bone loss and reduce the risk of fractures.

PRIMARY HYPERPARATHYROIDISM. Primary hyperparathyroidism occurs when one of our four parathyroid glands begins to produce too much parathyroid hormone (PTH). This is often the result of a noncancerous tumor known as an adenoma affecting the gland. Parathyroid hormone (not to be confused with thyroid hormone) helps the body tightly regulate the amount of calcium in the bloodstream – which is important for a number of essential body functions. Under normal circumstances, if blood calcium drops below its normal range, PTH is released to pull calcium from the bones to restore normal blood calcium levels. However, primary hyperparathyroidism causes a disconnection between the blood calcium levels and PTH – to the point where PTH is released even if blood calcium levels are normal or high! Excessive PTH stimulates osteoclasts to increase bone breakdown which elevates blood calcium levels beyond the normal limits (hypercalcemia). This can cause bones to become brittle.[27] Most of the time, this process does not cause any recognizable physical symptoms – however, severe hyperparathyroidism may cause bone pain, kidney stones, muscle aches, and mental disease.[28] Treatments including medication or surgery can reverse bone loss and reduce the risk of fractures. **If your head hurts trying to follow all of the information above, just remember that primary hyperparathyroidism leads to calcium being pulled from your bones, which weakens them over time and leads to osteoporosis!**

IDIOPATHIC HYPERCALCIURIA. Idiopathic hypercalciuria is when you pee out too much calcium (or, more technically, the excessive release of calcium in the urine without an identifiable underlying cause.) As one of my college professors once said, idiopathic means that we are "idiots" and "pathetic," and that's why we don't quite know the cause just yet. Patients with idiopathic hypercalciuria generally do not report any symptoms, however, a small percentage of patients do experience recurrent kidney stones. It has been shown that urinating high amounts of calcium over an extended period of time can weaken bones and increase the risk for fractures.[29] Unfortunately no cure currently exists. However, use of medications (including thiazide diuretics) may reduce the amount of calcium excreted in the urine and improve bone density.[30]

PRIMARY AND SECONDARY MALE HYPOGONADISM. **Primary hypogonadism** is a decrease in the amount of the hormone testosterone produced by the male testicles due to a disease within the testicles. **Secondary hypogonadism** refers to when the testicles do not receive the necessary chemical message from the brain to produce testosterone, leading to a reduction in testosterone levels. Men may experience several nonspecific symptoms including decreased libido, infertility, decreased testicular size, decreased energy, and decreased body hair. Both primary and secondary hypogonadism are significant risk factors for decreased bone density and fragility fractures in men because low testosterone levels can affect peak bone mass accrual and maintenance of bone strength.[31] Supplementing testosterone can improve bone density and decrease fracture risk in men with hypogonadism.

CELIAC DISEASE. Celiac disease is an autoimmune disorder in which the body's immune system produces antibodies to the gluten in our diet. These antibodies cause inflammation and irritation of the small intestine. Patients may be experience no symptoms with more mild forms of the disease, or may experience significant abdominal pain, chronic diarrhea, and unexplained weight loss after eating food containing gluten. Chronic inflammation of the small intestine can lead to poor absorption of essential bone building nutrients including calcium and vitamin D. Only 0.2% of the general population has celiac disease, however, 3.4% of patients with osteoporosis have the disease – indicating that it is a strong risk factor for developing osteoporosis.[32] Following a gluten free diet can improve the body's ability to absorb calcium and vitamin D, which may strengthen bones over time.

MULTIPLE MYELOMA. Multiple myeloma is a rare form of blood cancer. It affects the plasma cells produced in our bone marrow, which are responsible for key functions in our immune system. Most importantly, plasma cells make antibodies to fight infections. When a patient has multiple myeloma, the bone marrow produces too much of a single type of antibody. Because so much effort is put into making this one antibody, the body has less time and resources to produce other important blood cells. Initially, patients may not experience any symptoms, but in later stages patients may experience weight loss, frequent infections, bone pain, and fractures – particularly those involving the spine and ribs. Myeloma cells release chemicals which can break down bone and decrease new bone formation. Overall, this causes an increased risk of osteoporosis and fragility fractures.[33,34] Treatment by a blood cancer specialist would potentially include chemotherapy, radiation, stem cell transplant, and use of specific osteoporosis medications to decrease the risk of fracture.

CUSHING'S SYNDROME. Cushing's syndrome is caused by the excessive production of the hormone cortisol by the adrenal glands. Often times, this is caused by a benign tumor of the adrenal glands called an adenoma. Patients with Cushing's syndrome may experience a variety of symptoms including fatty deposits around the face and upper back (the so-called "humpback"), muscular weakness, easy bruising, high blood pressure, diabetes, and high cholesterol. Similar to patients taking steroid medications for long periods of time, prolonged exposure to cortisol and other steroid hormones can lead to increased bone breakdown, decreased bone formation and a rapid and profound decrease in bone strength. Treating the underlying cause of the condition with medication or surgery can improve bone density and decrease the risk of fragility fractures.

SYSTEMIC MASTOCYTOSIS. Systemic mastocytosis is the abnormal development of mast cells in multiple tissues throughout the body. Mast cells release chemical messages, including histamine, which serve an important role in allergic reactions. Patients may exhibit symptoms including abdominal pain, acid reflux, abnormal itchiness, anaphylactic (life-threatening) allergic reactions, and bone pain. Approximately 50% of patients with systemic mastocytosis will have bone problems including osteoporosis due to increased bone resorption.[35,36] No cure for systemic mastocytosis is currently available, but medications can reduce the unpleasant symptoms. If osteoporosis develops, specific osteoporosis medications will be required to improve bone density and decrease fracture risk.

What medications can cause secondary osteoporosis?

AROMATASE INHIBITORS (ANASTRAZOLE, LETROZOLE, EXEMESTRANE). Aromatase inhibitors are a class of chemotherapy medications used in women with breast and ovarian cancer. Many forms of breast and ovarian cancer are "estrogen receptor positive," meaning estrogen stimulates the growth and spread of these tumors. Aromatase inhibitors block the function of an enzyme called aromatase, which converts certain hormones into estrogen. As a result, aromatase inhibitors decrease the amount of estrogen available to fuel the growth of breast and ovarian tumors. As you might expect, this sudden decrease in estrogen has a similar effect on bone health as menopause. There is increased bone loss, decreased bone mineral density, and an increased fracture risk while taking these medications.[37,38]

ANTIDEPRESSANTS (SERTRALINE, CITALOPRAM, PAROXETINE, FLUOXETINE). Selective serotonin reuptake inhibitors (SSRIs) are the most popularly prescribed class of medications used to treat depression and anxiety disorders. Chemical messengers known as neurotransmitters allow nerve cells in the brain to communicate with one another. SSRIs work by increasing the chemical messenger serotonin in regions of the brain that control mood. This increased serotonin amplifies messages between nerve cells and ultimately leads to improved mood for those suffering from depression. SSRIs have also been shown to decrease the bone building osteoblasts activity and when compared to the general population, those taking SSRIs have a 1.6-fold greater rate of bone loss.[39,40]

ANTI-SEIZURE MEDICATIONS (CARBAMAZEPINE, VALPROATE, PHENOBARBITAL, PHENYTOIN). Anti-epileptic medications are a class of medications commonly used to treat seizures, and more recently, they have been used to stabilize mood in patients with bipolar disorder and other mood disorders. Anti-seizure medications work by making certain cells within the motor cortex (the part of the brain responsible for movement) less sensitive to chemical messages. This reduces the risk of unwanted movements, particularly seizures. These medications have been shown to decrease the availability of vitamin D and other nutrients which are necessary to maintain bone health. They are also associated with increased bone loss, decreased bone mineral density, and a 2 to 6-fold increase in fracture risk compared to the general population.[41-43]

CALCINEURIN INHIBITORS (CYCLOSPORIN, TACROLIMUS). Calcineurin inhibitors (CIs) are commonly used in patients after receiving an organ transplant to prevent rejection of the new organ. These medications inhibit the activity of a white blood cell involved in our immune response known as the T-lymphocyte. In doing so, the body is less likely to recognize the new organ as foreign and therefore less likely to reject the new organ. Calcineurin inhibitors have been associated with increased bone breakdown and decreased bone density.[44] One study showed that nearly 60% of patients taking CIs experienced a fracture within 6.5 years of receiving an organ transplant![45]

DEPOT MEDROXYPROGESTERONE ACETATE (DMPA). DMPA is form of female contraceptive that is administered via intra-muscular injection. The medication works by inhibiting the release of certain hormones (gonadotropins) from the pituitary gland in the brain. Decreased levels of gonadotropins prevent the female egg from being released by the ovaries (ovulation) and thicken the mucus in the cervix. This minimizes the chances of becoming pregnant. It is also associated with increased bone loss and decreased bone density – particularly in women older than 30 years of age who have received 10 or more DMPA injections in their lifetime.[46,47]

GNRH AGONISTS (LEUPRORELIN, TRIPTORELIN, GOSERELIN). GnRH agonists are commonly used in men with prostate cancer and women suffering from endometriosis. These medications suppress the chemical message that stimulates men to produce testosterone and women to produce estrogen. Decreased testosterone and estrogen have both been associated with worsening bone health and osteoporosis. GnRH agonists increase bone loss and decrease bone density. Prostate cancer patients treated with GnRH agonists have up to a 60% increased risk of fracture compared to the general population.[48]

PROTON PUMP INHIBITORS (OMEPRAZOLE, PANTOPRAZOLE). Proton pump inhibitors (PPIs) are commonly used for the treatment of acid reflux disease, stomach ulcers, and inflammation of the stomach (gastritis). PPIs decrease the amount of acid secretion in the stomach. Prolonged periods of acid suppression may impair the absorption of calcium and other important nutrients necessary for maintaining bone health. There is a modest association between the use of PPIs and an increased risk of hip and vertebral fractures.[49]

THIAZOLIDINEDIONES (ROSIGLITAZONE). Thiazolidinediones are used for the treatment of Type 2 diabetes. This medication increases the body's sensitivity to insulin, which decreases blood sugar levels and allows the body to use this sugar as a source of energy. Thiazolidinediones have been shown to decrease the activity of osteoblasts, leading to a decreased rate of new bone formation and increased fracture risk in people taking the medication.[50,51]

GLUCOCORTICOIDS (PREDNISONE, METHYLPREDNISOLONE). Glucocorticoids are commonly referred to as steroids. These medications are used to treat a wide variety of diseases, including those which cause severe inflammation, as well as those in which the body inappropriately produces antibodies against its own tissues (autoimmune disease). Of all the medications listed, steroids are the worst offenders when it comes to bone health. They present a double whammy by decreasing new bone formation AND increasing the breakdown of bone. Bone loss is rapid within the first 3-6 months of starting steroids, and an estimated 30-50% of patients on long-term glucocorticoids will break a bone at some point.[52,53] Steroids taken by mouth are worse for your bones than inhaled and topical forms of steroids, particularly when the daily dose is 5mg or greater for 3 months or longer. If your medical provider recommends that you take steroid medications for a prolonged period of time, discuss your risk of developing osteoporosis and what measures can be taken to minimize your risk of fractures.

Key Points

- Many medical diseases and commonly prescribed medications have been shown to increase the rate of bone loss and predispose patients to the development of osteoporosis.
- Treatment of patients with secondary osteoporosis is first aimed at treating the underlying condition, which may reverse bone loss and eliminate the need for other osteoporosis treatments. In other instances, no cure or medication alternative is available and osteoporosis specific treatments must be considered.
- If you have experienced any symptoms of the medical conditions listed above, or if you have taken any of the medications listed above, discuss your risk of developing osteoporosis with your medical provider.

3 | Screening for Osteoporosis: Pictures, Poking, and Prodding

Why screen for osteoporosis?

Osteoporosis is a silent disease – meaning that people with osteoporosis generally do not experience any physical symptoms. Patients do not call the doctor's office complaining of debilitating bone pain or a sensation of weak bones. Unless, of course, they just broke a bone… ouch! What makes osteoporosis scary is that people do not have any aggravating symptoms which serve as a motivator to be screened for the disease. Much like a heart attack may be the initial presentation of underlying heart disease; a fracture is often the initial presentation of a patient with osteoporosis – and at that point, we were too late! Medical providers screen for osteoporosis in an attempt to diagnose patients before significant bone loss has occurred. When osteoporosis is caught early, we can recommend lifestyle changes and other treatments to minimize the risk of fractures. The impact of fractures cannot be understated. While some are relatively minor and only require a short period of immobilization and physical therapy, others are debilitating and even life threatening. All too often, fractures permanently decrease a patient's quality of life. So why screen for osteoporosis? Hopefully the answer to this question is obvious by now, but screening is performed to identify high risk patients for osteoporosis! We can then start appropriate osteoporosis treatments to prevent fractures from occurring.

Who should be screened for osteoporosis?

The simple answer to the question "who should be screened for osteoporosis?" is that all men and women at increased risk for fracture should be screened. In reality, identifying these high risk patients isn't nearly as simple as it may sound. The only population that currently undergoes routine screening is **women over the age of 65**. The remainder of patients who are screened for osteoporosis are selected based on risk factors for fracture. With our current medical culture, it is not uncommon for high risk patients to slip through the cracks and never receive the screening they deserve. Below is a list of risk factors that should prompt a medical provider to evaluate a patient for osteoporosis. If any of these pertain to you, consider contacting your medical provider's office to schedule an osteoporosis evaluation.

FRAGILITY FRACTURES. People with hip, pelvis, spine, shoulder, or wrist fractures that result from low-energy trauma (including a fall from standing height) should be evaluated for osteoporosis. This is time sensitive as people are 86% more likely to sustain a second fracture in the twelve months following the initial fragility fracture compared to people with osteoporosis who have not broken a bone. With appropriate screening and treatment, the risk of sustaining a second fracture can be significantly reduced.

RADIOGRAPHIC OSTEOPENIA. In patients with osteoporosis, it is possible that a routine x-ray will raise suspicion for osteoporosis. It may come as a bit of a surprise when you go to your doctor's office for knee pain and the x-ray shows arthritis… and concern for osteoporosis. The bigger concern to you may be the knee pain, after all that is what caused you to schedule the appointment in the first place! But if your doctor recommends that you be screened for osteoporosis, take this recommendation seriously. While we cannot diagnose osteoporosis based on x-rays alone, the appearance of your bones on standard x-rays can raise suspicion for osteoporosis.

LOSS OF HEIGHT. Have you noticed that you are "shrinking" as you age, or that you are developing a "humpback?" It could be a sign that you have osteoporosis. People who are 1.5 inches shorter now compared to their peak adult height should be screened for osteoporosis. That "humpback" that you noticed could be the result of multiple compression fractures in your spine. It may appear to be just a cosmetic nuisance, but over time, it can significantly affect your balance and ability to breathe. Losing height and a change in the alignment of your back are not necessarily just a normal part of aging, so don't take them lightly!

BARIATRIC SURGERY AND MALABSORPTION. Surgeries that involve "shrinking" the stomach or removing a portion of the stomach/intestines, along with medical conditions including Celiac disease, can increase your risk of developing osteoporosis. These conditions make it more difficult for the body to absorb essential nutrients for maintaining strong bones. While no standardized recommendations are available for osteoporosis screening in patients with malabsorption, do not be surprised if your doctor suggests that you be screened.

USE OF MEDICATIONS ASSOCIATED WITH SECONDARY OSTEOPOROSIS. In the previous section I discussed several medications that are associated with secondary osteoporosis. The two biggest offenders are steroids and chemotherapy. The other medications listed in the previous section should be acknowledged by your medical provider; however, steroids and chemotherapy require more urgent evaluation for osteoporosis due to their dramatic negative impact on bone health.

CURRENT MEDICAL DIAGNOSIS ASSOCIATED WITH SECONDARY OSTEOPOROSIS. In the previous section I provided a detailed overview of medical diseases which are associated with developing osteoporosis. If you have ever been diagnosed with any of these conditions, your medical provider will recommend osteoporosis screening.

How are patients screened for osteoporosis?

A thorough screening for osteoporosis consists of three key components: the patient history, blood and/or urine labs, and the DXA bone density scan. None of these components are more important than the others, and all of these are crucial for managing the disease. If your medical provider says, "Let's just get a DXA scan to check your bones," don't accept this superficial screening. You and your bones deserve better than this lazy approach. Many factors go into determining what treatment plan is right for you, and the foundation for successful treatment begins with a comprehensive screening. Let's take a closer look at the key components of an osteoporosis evaluation.

- **PATIENT HISTORY.** Your provider should ask you a series of questions to identify risk factors associated with the development of osteoporosis and those which increase the risk of sustaining fractures. Topics will include your personal medial history, family history, and your lifestyle. You can find a list of questions that I use to screen patients in chapter 15.

- **DXA BONE DENSITY SCAN.** You will be sent for a DXA scan which provides a detailed analysis of your bone density. Continue on to the next section to learn more about DXA scans!

- **BLOOD AND/OR URINE LABS.** Following your appointment, you will be sent to the lab for blood tests, and sometimes even a urine test. These tests are used to ensure that key bone building nutrients are within normal ranges, as well as to screen for secondary causes of osteoporosis.

What is a DXA scan?

Dual-energy x-ray absorptiometry, more commonly known as a DXA scan, is a specialized x-ray of the hip, spine, or forearm used to measure bone density. Your medical provider will order a DXA scan of at least two locations in the body, most commonly the lower back and hip, to determine your bone density. In certain situations, including a history of a prior hip or back surgery with implanted metal, or prostate cancer in men, your doctor may include a DXA scan of the forearm for more accurate results.

How do I interpret my DXA scan results?

DXA scans allow for the measurement of bone density – that is, the amount of bone present in a specified amount of space. With DXA scans, density is a measurement of the number of grams of bone present in each square centimeter of a bone. Based on years of research, professionals in the field have determined the "normal" or "average" bone density of a healthy young adult between the ages of 25 and 35 with a low risk of sustaining a fracture. When a patient has a DXA scan, their personal bone density is compared to the bone density of the "normal" young adult and a number is generated, called a **T-score**. The T-score is used to categorize patients by their risk of sustaining a fracture. The further a patient's T-score is from normal, the greater the risk of breaking bones.

- **NORMAL BONE MINERAL DENSITY:** T-score +1.0 to -0.9
- **LOW BONE MINERAL DENSITY (OSTEOPENIA):** T-score -1.0 to -2.4
- **OSTEOPOROSIS:** T-score less than or equal to -2.5

Let's take a closer look at how to interpret T-scores. When a person's **bone density is exactly the same** as the normal young adult bone density, this would generate a T-score of 0. If a patient's **bone is STRONGER** than the normal young adult bone density, this would generate a T-score with a positive number. If a patient's **bone is WEAKER** than the normal young adult bone density, this would generate a T-score with a negative number. The further the number is from 0, the more significant the difference is between a patient's bone density and the normal young adult bone density. **More positive numbers correspond to increased bone density compared to normal, and more negative numbers correspond to decreased bone density compared to normal.**

Without considering any other factors (and we know there are many!), we can still roughly estimate your fracture risk based on your T-score value alone. As a rule of thumb, your fracture risk doubles with each single digit drop in T-score values below zero. A patient with a T-score of -1.0 has a 2-fold greater risk of fracture compared to a T-score of 0. Likewise, a T-score of -2.0 carries a 4-fold greater risk of fracture compared to a T-score of 0.

This concept may seem confusing if you are reading about it for the first time, so if your head is spinning, you are probably not alone! How about we consider an example? Let's compare patients with T-scores of -0.5 and -2.5. Both patients in this example have a negative T-score value, meaning their bone density is LESS than normal. The patient with the T-score of -0.5 is closer to zero, which means their bone density is closer to that of the normal young adult when compared to the patient with the T-score of -2.5. This means the patient with the T-score of -2.5 has a much LOWER bone density compared to the patient with the T-score of -0.5. If we look at the numbers listed above, the patient with the T-score of -2.5 would be classified as having osteoporosis, while the patient with the T-score of -0.5 would be classified has having "normal" bone density.

To complicate matters, there are a few quirks of DXA scans that need to be considered when interpreting your DXA results. When your doctor discusses your T-score, they will mention only a single number. However, if you look at the radiologist report from the scan, there are actually multiple T-scores listed! Each vertebra in the spinal column and different regions of the hip may have different T-score values. It is not uncommon to have significant differences between these numbers… so what leads to these differences and how do you know which number to use?

- **REASONS FOR FALSELY ELEVATED T-SCORES.** In the spine, there are many factors which may falsely increase the T-score. As we age, we are more likely to develop arthritis. With severe arthritis, bone spurs (osteophytes) may make the bones appear denser than they truly are. Compression fractures, which you now know are an indicator of osteoporosis, ironically may compress the bone and make it appear denser on the DXA scan! The DXA scanner may also pick up calcified blood vessels which overlap the spine and confuse this for calcification within the vertebrae. Finally, if a DXA scan is performed in a region that has metal hardware from a prior surgery, the results will be greatly altered. If your T-score is

+200, you are not superman, you probably just have metal plates or screws affecting your results!

- **REASONS FOR FALSELY DECREASED T-SCORES.** If the patient is rotated on the imaging table so that the x-ray image is no longer a straight on view of the spine, this may decrease how dense the bones appear.

When your medical provider receives the DXA report, they will closely review the results. Now… what to do about all of those T-scores? The current recommendation is to use the **lowest** T-score from the spine and/or hip when diagnosing osteoporosis.[54] For example, if a patient had a T-score of -2.3 at the hip and -2.6 at the L2 level of the spine, the T-score that would be used for diagnostic purposes would be -2.6, and the patient would be considered to have osteoporosis.

Now that you are familiar with T-scores, let's complicate matters even further by introducing the concept of a **Z-score**. If you recall, the T-score is a comparison of a patient's bone density to the bone density of a normal young adult. A Z-score, on the other hand, is a **comparison of a patient's bone density to the bone density of patient's just like them!** That is – patient's that are the same age, gender, and ethnicity. As we age, we would expect that our T-score would gradually get further away from the average young adult bone density because we slowly lose bone density after 30 years of age under normal circumstances. However, we would expect that our Z-score would stay close to the Z-scores of patients of the same age and gender because they are slowly losing bone density as well. If there is a substantial discrepancy in Z-scores, meaning that your bone density is significantly less than the density of other patients of similar age and ethnicity, this would raise suspicion that you might have a secondary cause of osteoporosis. In this scenario, further diagnostic screening is required to ensure no other factors are contributing to bone loss. Z-scores are also useful in helping medical providers identify high risk patients for osteoporosis in younger populations, including premenopausal women and men younger than 50 years old.

When should I have another DXA scan?

The interval of time between your initial DXA screening and a follow up DXA depends on the results of the initial scan.[55] In some instances, a follow up DXA scan may be warranted as often as yearly or every other year for close observation of your bone health. In others, you may not need another scan for a decade or longer! Below I will discuss how often a patient should have an updated DXA based on the T-score value of their scan.

- **T-SCORE LESS THAN -2.5.** If a patient has confirmed osteoporosis, the recommendation is to repeat the DXA scan every 2 years to monitor progression of the disease and/or response to osteoporosis treatment.

- **T-SCORE -2.0 TO -2.49 OR RISK FACTORS FOR ONGOING BONE LOSS.** If a patient has a high risk for developing osteoporosis in the near future, the recommendation is to repeat the DXA scan every 2 years.

- **T-SCORE -1.50 TO -1.99 AND NO RISK FACTORS FOR ACCELERATED BONE LOSS.** If a patient has a moderate risk for developing osteoporosis in the near future, the recommendation is to repeat the DXA scan in 3-5 years.

- **T-SCORE 0 TO -1.49 AND NO RISK FACTORS FOR ACCELERATED BONE LOSS.** If a patient has a low risk for developing osteoporosis in the near future, the recommendation is to repeat the DXA scan in 10-15 years.

What lab tests will my provider order… and why?

We all know that DXA scans are important in determining the density of bones, but no osteoporosis screening is complete without lab tests. So what labs come to mind? Calcium? Vitamin D? Those are certainly important. However, there are many others that are equally important. Your medical provider will order a series of blood and possibly even urine tests during a routine evaluation for osteoporosis. Below is a list of commonly ordered labs, as well as an explanation as to how these labs relate to your bone health.

COMPLETE BLOOD COUNT (CBC). The CBC is a measure of the different types of cells present within the blood; the most relevant to osteoporosis is hemoglobin. Low hemoglobin levels are commonly referred to as anemia. Patients may have anemia from simple causes such as iron deficiency, but it may also reflect less common underlying medical conditions including celiac disease, inflammatory disorders (e.g. rheumatoid arthritis), and even blood cancers such as multiple myeloma – all of which are known secondary causes of osteoporosis. If your CBC results show low levels of hemoglobin that are not explained by iron deficiency or other common causes, expect your medical provider to investigate further with other lab tests to evaluate for possible secondary causes of osteoporosis.

COMPREHENSIVE METABOLIC PANEL (CMP). The CMP is a combination of labs, all of which relate to metabolism. Our metabolism is the series of chemical reactions that keeps our bodies ticking. This panel includes a measure of kidney and liver function, important electrolytes including calcium and phosphorus, and blood sugar levels. Kidney and liver disease can affect how the body processes calcium, phosphorus, vitamin D, and other key contributors to bone health. Calcium is arguably the most important mineral in building bone density, but don't confuse a normal calcium lab result with good bone health. If we do not consume enough calcium through our diet, the body will pull it from our bones in order to maintain blood calcium levels in the normal range. As you can imagine, this negatively impacts bone density. Finally, the CMP measures blood sugar levels. Elevated blood sugars on an empty stomach indicate diabetes, which is also a known risk factor for osteoporosis and fractures.

25-HYDROXYVITAMIN D. Vitamin D is found in many different forms within the body – the most meaningful and commonly measured when it comes to osteoporosis is 25-hydroxyvitamin D. Vitamin D is important for calcium absorption in our intestines. Low levels of vitamin D will significantly reduce the amount of calcium absorbed from the dairy, green leafy vegetables, and fortified cereals in our diet. Over time, this can predispose a patient to osteoporosis. It is important that your medical provider makes sure that your vitamin D levels are within the normal range before considering the different treatment options for osteoporosis. Failure to do so can lead to unpleasant side effects which are entirely preventable.

PARATHYROID HORMONE (PTH). You learned in the section discussing secondary causes of osteoporosis that parathyroid hormone helps the body regulate the amount of calcium in the bloodstream. If you recall, people with hyperparathyroidism have a noncancerous tumor in the parathyroid gland which causes increased PTH levels even when there is already enough calcium in the bloodstream, leading to bones become progressively more brittle because PTH is constantly leeching calcium from the bones.

For this reason, a lab test which measures your parathyroid hormone level is commonly included in a screening for osteoporosis. People with hyperparathyroidism will have high levels of parathyroid hormone, as well as high levels of calcium in their bloodstream.

THYROID STIMULATING HORMONE (TSH). Thyroid hormone has a number of roles within the body including regulation of vital functions such as heart rate and breathing. It also influences the rate of our metabolism. High levels of thyroid hormone, as indicated by a low TSH lab value, are a known risk factor for accelerated bone loss.

24-HOUR URINE CALCIUM. The 24-hour urine calcium lab is just as the name implies – it is a measure of the amount of calcium that is released in the urine over a 24 hour period of time. A small amount of calcium in the urine is normal, but abnormally high amounts can affect bone health. A medical condition known as idiopathic hypercalciuria (meaning too much calcium is released in the urine for no known reason) can predispose a patient to osteoporosis. If you have a history of kidney stones, or if your medical provider is concerned about the possibility of secondary osteoporosis, do not be surprised if this test is ordered.

TISSUE TRANSGLUTAMINASE ANTIBODY (TTG). In patients with celiac disease, the body's immune system creates antibodies to gluten in the diet. Over time, these antibodies can damage the lining of our intestines, which can affect our ability to absorb key nutrients including calcium and vitamin D. A measurement of one such antibody, known as tTG, is used to determine if a patient has celiac disease. The disease can negatively impact bone density if left untreated. Those who follow a gluten free diet will improve the ability of the intestines to absorb key nutrients and even improve bone density.

SERUM/URINE PROTEIN ELECTROPHORESIS. Serum/urine protein electrophoresis is a test reserved for patients that demonstrate risk factors for multiple myeloma – a rare form of blood cancer which can lead to a rapid loss of bone density. If you have experienced unexplained anemia (especially if combined with low white blood cell and platelet counts), weight loss, bone pain, or fractures, your medical provider will likely order this test.

SALIVARY CORTISOL. The hormone cortisol is generally measured through a noninvasive sampling of our saliva. Cortisol is commonly referred to as the "stress hormone" and has important roles relating to metabolism and the immune system. This lab value provides a fairly crude measurement of cortisol levels because there is significant variability in cortisol throughout the day. However, if levels are elevated (a medical condition known as Cushing's syndrome), this could be an indication of a tumor in the adrenal glands which can lead to weakened bones.

FASTING MORNING TESTOSTERONE, LH/FSH. Men with osteoporosis frequently have low levels of testosterone (hypogonadism). Symptoms of hypogonadism are quite subjective – decreased libido, low energy – but if these are present in men with osteoporosis, your medical provider may recommend a blood test to check testosterone levels. Select men may benefit from supplementation of testosterone to improve their bone density if hypogonadism is present.

One last lab… measuring bone turnover markers.

Bone turnover markers (BTMs) are chemical byproducts of bone remodeling – which is the process of old bone being recycled and new, healthy bone being formed in its place. This process is completely normal and constantly occurring throughout the skeletal system. However, the rate of remodeling can speed up or slow down over time. Three commonly measured markers are released into the bloodstream during this process and provide an estimation of the rate of bone remodeling. BTMs are helpful in monitoring response to osteoporosis treatments, as the treatments available will impact the rate of remodeling. It is important to understand that bone turnover markers have no use in the diagnosis of osteoporosis, but they are useful for monitoring your response to treatment over time.

Should I have my BTMs checked?

Not all people with osteoporosis need to have their bone turnover markers checked. The initial lab value isn't all that useful in isolation because the number can vary so significantly from one person to the next. Bone turnover markers ARE useful in **monitoring a person's response to osteoporosis medication over time.** People who are considering osteoporosis medications may have their BTMs measured just before the start of taking a new medication, and again **3-6 months** later. Depending on the type of medication, we would expect the BTM labs to either increase or decrease by a certain amount to determine how well the medication is working. This provides a reasonably quick confirmation that the medication is doing its job – instead of waiting for a DXA scan which takes **2 years** to show significant improvement in bone density. Two years can feel like an eternity when it comes to improving your bone health! BTMs are particularly useful in high risk patients including those with severe osteoporosis, those with a condition known to cause malabsorption of key nutrients, or those with prior surgery involving the stomach/intestines. Below you will find more detailed information regarding common BTMs.[56-58]

SERUM C-TERMINAL TELOPEPTIDE OF TYPE I COLLAGEN (CTX). CTX is measured in the blood and indicates the rate of bone resorption (recycling). If a person is responding appropriately to treatment, we would expect this lab value to decrease by 30% 3-6 months following the start of treatment.

URINARY N-TERMINAL TELOPEPTIDE OF TYPE I COLLAGEN (NTX). NTX is measured in the urine and indicates the rate of bone resorption (recycling). If a patient is responding appropriately to treatment, we would expect this lab value to decrease by 50% 3-6 months following the start of treatment.

SERUM TYPE I PROCOLLAGEN N-TERMINAL (PINP). P1NP is measured in the blood and indicates the rate of bone formation (bone building). If a patient is responding appropriately to treatment, we would expect this lab value to increase by at least 21% 3-6 months following the start of treatment.

Key Points

- Screening for osteoporosis consists of a thorough patient history, blood and/or urine labs, and a DXA bone density scan.
- All women over the age of 65 should be screened for osteoporosis. Women younger than 65 years old and men should be screened based on the presence of risk factors for osteoporosis.
- DXA scans are specialized x-rays of the hip, spine, and forearm used to determine the density of bones, measured in grams per square centimeter.
- A number of different labs may be ordered to ensure adequate levels of calcium and vitamin D. The labs will also assess for secondary causes of osteoporosis, which require specific treatment considerations that are different than the traditional treatments for osteoporosis.

- Bone turnover markers may be used to monitor response to treatment over time, but are not used to diagnose osteoporosis.

I have been questioned, scanned, poked, and prodded… now what?

As you know, people are more than just T-scores and lab values. The sole purpose of screening for osteoporosis isn't to label you with a number, but to determine your risk of sustaining a fracture. We do not treat numbers, though these numbers do provide useful information. Once all of the necessary information has been gathered, your medical provider will calculate your risk of sustaining a fracture in the future and determine which treatment options are best for you!

How is my fracture risk calculated?

The most important step in managing osteoporosis is determining each person's individualized risk of breaking a bone. Contrary to what you may have been told, not all people with the same T-scores have the same risk of fracturing – there are many other variables that need to be considered. For example, let us compare a 50 year old and 80 year old with the same T-score of -2.5. Both would be diagnosed as having osteoporosis, however, the 80 year old has a 5-fold higher risk of sustaining a fracture compared to the 50 year old patient![59] These two patients may require vastly different treatments even though their T-scores are identical!

Now let's consider another example with two 65 year old female patients. The first patient has a T-score of -2.5, indicating the presence of osteoporosis. The second patient has a T-score of -2.0, indicating low bone mineral density (osteopenia), but without osteoporosis. However, the patient without osteoporosis does have other risk factors including smoking, a prior fracture, and a family history of osteoporosis fractures. Even though this patient doesn't have osteoporosis based on their T-score value, their risk of suffering a major osteoporosis fracture in the next 10 years is 3-fold higher than the patient with osteoporosis!

So how exactly do we calculate a patient's risk of fracturing in the future? The World Health Organization developed the Fracture Risk Assessment Tool (**FRAX**) which allows medical providers to calculate each patient's 10 year risk of sustaining a hip or other major osteoporosis related fracture. The tool is useful for men and women between the ages of 40 and 90 years old. It takes into account multiple risk factors for osteoporosis, including age, weight, parental hip fracture, personal history of fragility fracture or secondary osteoporosis, tobacco and alcohol use, rheumatoid arthritis, steroid use, and the patient's hip T-score. Patients are considered high risk for fracture if their 10 year risk of a **hip fracture is greater than 3%,** or their 10 year risk for a **major osteoporosis related fracture (including hip, spine, wrist, shoulder, and pelvis fractures) is greater than 20%.** If you recently had a bone density scan, ask your medical provider to calculate your FRAX score and discuss your fracture risk with you.

It may seem like I have been recommending aggressive osteoporosis management for all high risk patients to minimize fracture risk… and I have been doing just that! But did you know that some people with confirmed osteoporosis (T-score less than -2.5) may not need any osteoporosis medications because their risk of fracture is actually quite low? You might be thinking to yourself "I thought ALL people with osteoporosis were high risk" but that isn't necessarily true. Certain fracture risk factors carry more weight than others. For example, the FRAX calculator only uses your hip T-score value because it is much more predictive of future fractures than your spine T-score value. That doesn't mean that the spine T-score isn't important… it absolutely is! But if a patient is relatively young with am osteoporotic spine T-score and only a mildly decreased hip T-score value, it is very reasonable to have your doctor monitor your bone density over time and recommend simple lifestyle changes as opposed to considering medications.

On the flipside, it is also possible that a patient that does not have osteoporosis (T-score greater than -2.5) WILL be recommended to take osteoporosis medication. If a patient has multiple risk factors for osteoporosis, a T-score outside of the osteoporosis range may still be associated with an unacceptably high fracture risk. Only after all variables are carefully considered should your medical provider recommend appropriate treatment options.

Key Points

- Multiple variables must be carefully considered when determining a patient's risk of fractures.
- The Fracture Risk Assessment Tool (FRAX) developed by the World Health Organization allows medical providers to calculate a

patient's 10 year risk of hip and major osteoporosis related fractures.

- High risk patients have a 10 year **hip fracture risk greater than 3%,** and/or a 10 year **major osteoporosis related fracture risk (including hip, spine, wrist, shoulder, and pelvis fractures) greater than 20%.**
- Your T-score should not be the only variable used to determine which treatment is best for you!

5 | Who Should be Considered for Treatment?

In previous chapters I have alluded to the fact that osteoporosis treatments are available to increase bone strength and decrease your risk of breaking bones. Certain treatment recommendations apply to everyone, whereas others are generally reserved for patients that have a significant risk of breaking bones. While there are no rigid guidelines as to which patients should to be treated, well respected medical organizations have proposed widely accepted recommendations which help to identify high risk patients that would benefit from osteoporosis treatment. You might be thinking, "Well, who are these people and how do I know if I'm one of them?" In this chapter I will discuss the men and women who qualify for osteoporosis treatment.

Which men should be considered for osteoporosis treatment?

Most people typically associate low bone density and osteoporosis with elderly women, but don't tell that to the 8 million men in the United States that are affected by the disease.[60] Men do not experience the menopause-induced loss of bone that plagues women – instead, under normal physiologic conditions there is a gradual loss of testosterone production and a slow decline in bone health. Because of this, men generally develop osteoporosis and fragility fractures 10 years later than women. This doesn't necessarily mean than men are off the hook until their 70s... As we explored earlier, up to 75% of men with osteoporosis have a secondary cause which can lead to fragility fractures well before that time.[61] To make matters worse, men tend to be more severely impaired following fragility fractures. While men account for 25% of hip fractures, they have a 2-fold greater risk of death following a hip fracture compared to their female counterparts.[62,63]

We have established that men carry a significant lifetime risk of developing osteoporosis and that the prognosis following fractures in men is often worse than that observed in women. This begs the question – which men should be considered for osteoporosis treatment? The first group is men with an **established diagnosis of osteoporosis**. The criteria used to diagnose osteoporosis in men vary based on the age of the individual.

- **MEN OLDER THAN 50 YEARS OF AGE.** Osteoporosis is defined as a T-score less than -2.5.[64]

- **MEN YOUNGER THAN 50 YEARS OF AGE.** Osteoporosis is defined as a Z-score less than -2.0 along with a history of a fragility fracture.[65]

Men without an established diagnosis of osteoporosis, but with **significant risk factors for fragility fracture**, may also be considered for osteoporosis treatment. Below is a list of risk factors that should prompt your medical provider to consider you for treatment.

- **FRAX SCORE.** Men of any age with a 10 year hip fracture risk greater than 3% or a 10 year major osteoporosis fracture risk greater than 20% should be considered for treatment.

- **FRAGILITY FRACTURE.** A prior fragility fracture, regardless of bone density, is a strong predictor of future fractures and should prompt consideration for osteoporosis treatment.

- **RISK FOR ACCELERATED BONE LOSS.** Patients with certain diseases or who take medications associated with accelerated bone loss are at increased risk of developing osteoporosis. Appropriate treatment must be considered in this patient population.

Which women should be considered for osteoporosis treatment?

Postmenopausal women are most commonly affected by osteoporosis due to the abrupt loss of over 10% of their bone density from estrogen deficiency following menopause. However, premenopausal women are at risk for developing osteoporosis as well. In general, women with **inadequate peak bone mass acquisition** during their teenage years are at increased risk developing osteoporosis at younger ages because their "stored bone" will not be able to withstand the gradual bone loss that occurs after age 30. Women with **ongoing accelerated bone loss** from a variety of underlying medical conditions or use of certain medications are also at increased risk for early osteoporosis.

Over 20 million women in the United States have low bone density and osteoporosis.[66] It has been shown that 30-40% of women older than 50 years of age will experience a fragility fracture during their lifetime.[67] Given the prevalence of the disease, and the pain and suffering that result from fractures, it is important to screen and appropriately treat women with osteoporosis or those at high risk of breaking bones.

The criteria used to diagnose osteoporosis in women vary based on the age of the patient because the relationship between bone density and fracture risk is not the same among premenopausal and postmenopausal women.

- **POSTMENOPAUSAL WOMEN.** Osteoporosis is defined as a T-score less than -2.5.[68]

- **PREMENOPAUSAL WOMEN.** Osteoporosis is defined as a Z-score less than -2.0 with a history of a fragility fracture.[69]

Women without an established diagnosis of osteoporosis, but with significant risk factors for fragility fracture, may also be considered for osteoporosis treatment. Below is a list of risk factors that should prompt consideration for osteoporosis treatment.

- **FRAX SCORE.** Women of any age with a 10 year hip fracture risk greater than 3%, or a 10 year major osteoporosis related fracture risk greater than 20% should be considered for treatment.

- **FRAGILITY FRACTURE.** A prior fragility fracture, regardless of bone density, is a strong predictor of future fractures and should prompt consideration for osteoporosis treatment.

- **RISK FOR ACCELERATED BONE LOSS.** Patients with certain diseases or who take medications associated with accelerated bone loss are at increased risk of developing osteoporosis. Appropriate treatment must be considered in this patient population.

Which patients taking oral steroids should be considered for osteoporosis treatment?

Approximately 1.2% of the population takes long term oral steroids; representing a small, but significant group of patients that are at increased risk of developing osteoporosis.[70] Those starting oral steroids experience a rapid loss of bone density within the first 3-6 months related to **increased bone resorption** and **decreased new bone formation.**[71] An estimated 30-50% of patients on chronic steroids will sustain a fracture at some point, and fractures can occur in patients with higher bone density than those sustained by the general population.[71,72] Since the spine has a higher proportion of cancellous bone which is very metabolically active and can change quickly, the negative effects of steroids typically show up here first. This makes patients particularly vulnerable to vertebral (spine) compression fractures.[73] Fracture risk varies with steroid dose and with the duration of treatment. Those taking high doses of steroids (greater than 5mg daily) for prolonged periods of time (longer than 3 months) have the greatest risk of fracture.[73] Following termination of the medication or with use of osteoporosis medications, patients can increase their bone density and decrease their fracture risk, however, an elevated risk of fracture may be premanent.[73]

Patients taking steroids require special consideration in regard to osteoporosis management and prevention because of the significant decrease in bone density and increase in fracture risk associated with these medications. This is why a separate section was provided to discuss osteoporosis treatment in those taking steroid medications! Below is a list of risk factors that should prompt consideration for osteoporosis treatment.[74-76]

- **ESTABLISHED DIAGNOSIS OF OSTEOPOROSIS.** All patients with an established diagnosis of osteoporosis, regardless of dose or duration of steroid treatment, should be considered for osteoporosis management while taking steroids.

- **FRAX SCORE.** A 10-year hip fracture risk greater than 3% or a 10 year major osteoporosis related fracture risk greater than 20% should prompt consideration for osteoporosis management, regardless of the T-score.

- **STEROID DOSE.** All patients (regardless of age and gender) taking steroids doses of at least 5mg daily for 3 or more months should be considered for osteoporosis management given the significant fracture risk with high doses of these medications.

- **PRIOR FRAGILITY FRACTURE.** All patients with a prior fragility fracture should be considered high risk for fracture while taking any dose of oral steroids.

- **ONGOING LOSS OF BONE MINERAL DENSITY.** It is recommended that all patients taking high doses of oral steroids have **yearly DXA scans** to evaluate for progression of osteoporosis. If the DXA scans show greater than 4% loss of bone mineral density 2 years in a row, the patient should be considered for osteoporosis management, regardless of their T-score.

6 | How to Evaluate which Treatments Actually Work?

It may seem daunting when you begin to research all of the available treatment options for osteoporosis. With all of the medications and recommendations, it can make your head spin! To complicate matters, authors of popular osteoporosis books and websites have often varied in their recommendations… so which treatment is right for you?

To answer this question, we need to look at the most unbiased source for accurate information – research studies performed at academic facilities. But don't be fooled! To the untrained eye, it is easy for an author to misconstrue the results of these studies to fit their own agenda, and unfortunately this runs rampant in osteoporosis texts and websites. You don't have to look far to find a sensationalized article promoting a brand new "natural" treatment, or a "proven" workout and diet that will reverse the disease. Throw in a good conspiracy theory regarding how medical providers are promoting "dangerous" and "ineffective" medications and you now have no idea what to think!

You might be thinking to yourself, "How am I supposed to find good research articles, and more importantly, how will I be able to interpret the results on my own?" This is a fair question. It is unfortunate that these articles are not always available for the general public to view, and when available, they are often filled with confusing and intimidating medical terminology that is difficult to understand. It is far more convenient to read an author's review of the research in patient-friendly language. The goal of this section is not to teach you how to understand every aspect of these research articles, but to help you identify which are high quality with meaningful results, and which you should question. Below is a list of terms and concepts that should be included in every high quality research study.

- **PLACEBO-CONTROLLED.** To ensure that any positive or negative result of the experiment did not occur simply due to chance, participants receiving a treatment need to be compared to a group receiving a placebo (this is generally a "fake" treatment or no treatment at all). If 10% of patients receiving a medication report stomach pain, it is tempting to call this a side effect of the medication. However, if 10% of the placebo patients experience the same stomach pain, it could be that stomach pain is just a common occurrence in day to day life and that the medication does not actually cause this side effect. Without proper comparison to a group receiving placebo, the results are incomplete and difficult to interpret.

- **RANDOMIZED.** To avoid bias, researchers must randomly assign study participants into the treatment group (the group receiving the medication or therapy) or the placebo group (the group receiving a fake treatment, or no treatment at all). If researchers did not use a randomized design and instead hand-selected particular patients for one treatment group or the other, this may alter the results of the experiment.

- **DOUBLE-BLIND.** A double blind study means that both the participants and the researchers measuring the results are unaware of which participants are receiving the treatment, and which are receiving the placebo. If an experiment is not double-blind, researchers are aware of the patients receiving treatment. If researchers are motivated for the experiment to find significant results, they may be biased in reporting positive outcomes in a particular group.

- **STATISTICAL SIGNIFICANCE.** Results of a study are said to be "statistically significant" if the data analysis shows the difference between the results in the treatment and placebo groups are so different that it is unlikely that the difference is due to chance. Results are said to be "not statistically significant" if a difference exists, but the difference is small and could be explained by chance. This is probably the most important concept of all! Not all results are statistically significant, regardless of what others may lead you to believe in their publications!

In order to make sure that the results are accurate and trustworthy, they should come from high quality randomized, double-blind, placebo-controlled research studies with statistically significant results! If the results come from poorly designed studies without a placebo control, then an appropriate statistical analysis cannot be performed to determine statistical significance and the results are fairly useless. Be sure to keep this concept in mind when evaluating osteoporosis treatment recommendations from other sources.

What treatment options are available for osteoporosis?

So without further ado, let's discuss the available treatment options. When I consider osteoporosis treatments, I divide them into two categories – the primary treatments and adjunct treatments. The primary treatments are those which have been proven to reduce a patient's risk of sustaining a fracture, whereas the adjunct treatments are those that improve bone health but have not been shown in scientific studies to reduce fracture risk on their own.

The primary treatment options for osteoporosis are the homerun hitters on the team. What sets these medications apart from the adjunct treatments is that they have been proven to reduce the risk of fracture between 50-75% in large scientific studies. On the other hand, adjunct treatments are the foundation for excellent bone health. They may slow the progression of the disease and in some instances even lead to a small increase in bone density. However, not all treatments that improve bone density have been shown to decrease the risk of sustaining a fracture – which is the primary reason that we treat osteoporosis! None of the adjunct treatments have been shown to decrease the risk of sustaining a fracture, but remain important in the management of osteoporosis. A thorough review of all treatment options will follow in the upcoming chapters. You should learn all of the necessary information and discuss all options with your medical provider before committing to any treatment plan.

ADJUNCT TREATMENTS FOR OSTEOPOROSIS

- WHOLE BODY VIBRATION THERAPY
- WEIGHT BEARING EXERCISE PROGRAM
- CALCIUM: 1200 MG DAILY
- VITAMIN D: 800 IU DAILY
- SMOKING CESSATION
- MODEST ALCOHOL CONSUMPTION (<2 ALCOHOLIC BEVERAGES DAILY)

PRIMARY TREATMENTS FOR OSTEOPOROSIS

- ESTROGEN/SELECTIVE ESTROGEN REUPTAKE MODULATORS
- BISPHOSPHONATES (FOSAMAX, ACTONEL, RECLAST)

- **DENOSUMAB (PROLIA)**
- **TERIPARATIDE (FORTEO)**

7 | Whole Body Vibration

What is whole body vibration?

Whole body vibration is a treatment used to manage osteoporosis in a manner that is exactly as it sounds – patients sit or stand on a device that sends waves of vibrations through the entire body. While this treatment is not approved by the Food and Drug Administration (FDA) for the treatment of osteoporosis, there have been several research studies performed in an effort to determine its effects on bone density and fractures. How exactly does whole body vibration work? This is a tricky question because the mechanism is not well understood. It is believed to stimulate the muscles and bones within the body, and in animal models it has been shown to stimulate the activity of the bone building osteoblast cells.[77]

Which features should you consider in a whole body vibration machine?

Many different models of vibration machines are currently available on the market. They vary significantly in the speed and intensity of vibration and there is no standardization by the FDA to regulate these variables. Vibration platforms are not covered by insurance companies and typically cost around $1600. The current recommendation from experienced sources is to use low intensity vibration platforms for 10 minutes daily.[77] Consider platforms with handrails and other safety features to minimize the risk of fall or injury during use.

What are possible side effects of whole body vibration?

A discussion of adverse events is not frequently included in any of the research studies that evaluate vibration machines, but that does not necessarily mean that this treatment is risk free. Use of vibrating machinery in the workforce has been associated with low back pain and muscle aches, problems with balance, dizziness, and episodes of low blood pressure. Sources familiar with the use of vibration platforms for osteoporosis have reported plantar fasciitis, itchiness, blurred vision, ringing in the ears, loss of balance and falls in patients using these devices.[77]

How effective is whole body vibration in treating osteoporosis?

Many studies have been performed throughout the years evaluating the effect of vibration machines on a variety of physical ailments. Several of these studies have been specifically designed to evaluate the effect of vibration platforms in patients with osteoporosis; however, most of these studies are poor quality. A meta-analysis (review of multiple research studies all examining the same treatment) which included twelve reasonably well designed studies comparing the effect of vibration platforms on bone density was reviewed.[77] Even in these studies, the researchers lacked standardization and varied significantly in their vibration protocols. The amount of time patients spent on the vibrating device was between 15 seconds to 30 minutes, and the frequency was between 1 to 7 days per week. In general, the lower the vibration intensity, the longer and more frequent the recommended treatments. Studies in the meta-analysis lasted from less than 1 year, to 7 years and longer. The results of this meta-analysis in regard to the effect of whole body vibration on bone density and fracture risk are discussed below.

BONE DENSITY AND FRACTURE RISK. Most studies reported a 1.5% to 4.3% increase in bone density of the spine and hip. These results were reported as insignificant by the researchers because they did not vary enough from the bone density of control patients who did not use vibration machines. Two of the 12 studies did report a significant increase in bone density at the hip, and 1 reported a significant increase at the spine. One study found a DECREASE in wrist bone density among patients using the vibration platform. It is safe to say that vibration machines may have a small positive impact on bone density. However, **none of the 12 studies found whole body vibration therapy to reduce the risk of sustaining a fracture** despite these small increases in bone density.

RESULTS AT A GLANCE	
DOES VIBRATION THERAPY IMPROVE BONE DENSITY?	Two of the twelve studies found a significant increase in bone density among patients using vibration therapy. Bone density increased between 1.5% and 4.3% in most patients.
DOES VIBRATION THERAPY DECREASE FRACTURE RISK?	No studies have shown vibration therapy to decrease the risk of sustaining fractures.

The bottom line on using whole body vibration to treat osteoporosis…

Whole body vibration is a treatment option that has not been approved by the FDA for the treatment of osteoporosis, but has been evaluated experimentally to determine the effects on bone density and fracture risk. This therapy involves the patient standing or sitting on a vibrating platform to stimulate bone and muscle. Overall, it has been shown to have a small positive effect on bone density, indicating that it may slow the progression of the disease. However, it has not been shown to decrease the risk sustaining a fracture and should not be the sole treatment for patients at high risk for fracture. Patients who are at low risk of fracture and those who wish to avoid medications can consider adding vibration therapy to a comprehensive treatment plan for optimal results.

8 | Weight Bearing Exercise

What is weight bearing exercise?

Weight bearing exercise has been proposed as an option for the treatment of osteoporosis. The definition of weight bearing exercise has proven to be quite variable from one source to the next. Some studies included simple exercises such as brisk walking, where others involved aerobic exercises and even heavy weightlifting programs.[78] It is thought that weight bearing exercise places stress across our bones – and in response, the bones adapt to the stress by becoming stronger. This is the same concept behind lifting weights to build larger and stronger muscles. Several studies have evaluated the effect of these various forms of weight bearing exercise on bone density and fracture risk, and these will be discussed below.

What are possible side effects of weight bearing exercise?

A discussion of adverse events was not included in the research studies that were reviewed, but that does not necessarily mean that this treatment is risk free. It is best to consult your medical provider before starting any new workout program, particularly if you have a history of heart disease or joint problems.

How effective is weight bearing exercise in treating osteoporosis?

A meta-analysis consisting of 18 well-designed clinical trials that were randomized and controlled to evaluate the effect of different weight bearing exercise programs was reviewed.[78] Three distinct forms of workout programs were evaluated – **aerobic exercise** consisting of calisthenics (bodyweight exercises), walking, stretching, and strengthening, **resistance training** consisting of a weightlifting program, and a **fast walking** program. Combined, these studies included 1423 postmenopausal women between the ages of 45 and 70. The studies ranged in length from as little as 8 weeks, to longer than 3 years and generally recommended that participants perform the physical activity at least 2 or 3 times weekly. The results of this meta-analysis in regard to the effect of weight bearing exercise on bone density and fracture risk are discussed below.

BONE DENSITY AND FRACTURE RISK. Aerobic exercise, resistance training, and fast walking were associated with a small improvement in bone density of the spine. Interestingly, aerobic exercise was the only form of exercise that improved bone density at the wrist, and fast walking was the only form of exercise that improved hip bone density. More recent studies have shown resistance training exercises may also have a small impact on hip bone density as well. **No studies have shown weight bearing exercise of any form to decrease the risk of sustaining a fracture, even in studies extending beyond 2 years.**

RESULTS AT A GLANCE	
DOES WEIGHT BEARING EXERCISE IMPROVE BONE DENSITY?	Fast walking and resistance training led to improvements in hip and spine bone density, whereas aerobic exercise led to an increase in spine and wrist bone density.
DOES WEIGHT BEARING EXERCISE DECREASE FRACTURE RISK?	No studies have shown weight bearing exercise to decrease the risk of sustaining fractures.

The bottom line on using weight bearing exercise to treat osteoporosis…

Weight bearing exercise includes a variety of workout programs which aim to stress the skeletal system and improve bone density. Proposed programs range from fast walking to structured weightlifting sessions. Overall, these have been shown to have a small positive effect on bone density, indicating that they may slow the progression of osteoporosis. However, no weight bearing exercise program has been shown to decrease the risk of sustaining a fracture. For now, this treatment option is best reserved as an adjunct to other treatments. Patients who are at low risk of fracture and those who wish to avoid medications should consider adding weight bearing exercise to a comprehensive treatment plan as it is a reasonably safe alternative that has health benefits extending beyond the skeletal system.

9 | Calcium and Vitamin D

Why is calcium important in osteoporosis care?

It would be a rare occurrence that you and your medical provider would have a conversation about osteoporosis without calcium being mentioned at least once. You may have even "had the talk" about getting adequate calcium through your diet and adding calcium supplements if needed. But why exactly is calcium important for bone health? Calcium is an essential nutrient that serves as the main building block in the structural integrity of bone.[79] It is the primary mineral component of bone with 99% of the body's calcium stored in bone tissue – and we want the calcium to remain stored there! If you fail to get enough calcium in your diet, your body will pull calcium from the bones to perform vital bodily functions that rely on this calcium. Over time, this can lead to brittle bones and fractures. Bottom line… calcium is critically important for good bone health!

What happens if I do not consume enough calcium in my diet?

I alluded to the answer of this question in prior sections, but let's take a closer look. Aside from calcium's role in maintaining bone density, it also serves a number of other critical functions. These include roles in muscle contraction, nerve impulses, blood clotting, and communication between body cells. In order to adequately perform these duties, calcium is maintained in our bloodstream at a level between 8.5 and 10.2 mg/dL. This level of calcium is primarily maintained by calcium consumed through our diet or by calcium supplements. If we do not consume enough calcium, the body looks to pull calcium from the next most logical place – our bones! The process is controlled by parathyroid hormone and is fairly complex, but the end result of prolonged calcium deficiency is decreased bone density and increased fracture risk.[80]

How much calcium should I consume each day?

The general recommendation for daily calcium intake among both men and women is **1200mg** daily.[81] The body can absorb about 500mg of calcium in one sitting, so it is best to split up your dairy intake or calcium supplements throughout the day. To minimize the possible side effects of calcium, avoid consuming greater than 2000mg daily, take calcium supplements with meals, and obtain at least 50% of your calcium intake from dietary sources!

How much calcium is in common dietary sources?

Calcium is found in a variety of food sources. Most people are aware that dairy products are rich in calcium, but you may not know that dark green vegetables, nuts, breads, and fortified cereals may also contain a significant amount of calcium as well! Below is a list representing the amount of calcium in common dietary sources. If after adding up your daily calcium you do not reach 1200mg, consider how you can increase calcium intake through your diet or through calcium supplements.

- **300MG PER SERVING**: 8ounces of milk or yogurt, 1ounce of hard cheese
- **150MG PER SERVING**: 4 ounces of cottage cheese or ice cream
- **100-200MG PER SERVING:** dark green vegetables, nuts, breads, soy beans, fortified cereals

Should I supplement with calcium carbonate or calcium citrate?

If you have gone shopping for calcium supplements recently, you may have discovered that two forms of calcium are readily available over the counter. So which is better? For most people, both calcium carbonate and calcium citrate would be a perfectly fine choice. The only exception is in people who take medications to reduce stomach acid (including Omeprazole and Ranitidine). If this applies to you, then calcium citrate is the preferred supplement because it is better absorbed in low-acidity environments.[82]

What are possible side effects of calcium supplementation?

As with all treatment options, no matter how natural or holistic they may appear, there is always a risk for side effects. In order to minimize the risk of adverse events, it is recommended that people obtain at least half of their calcium intake through dietary sources as opposed to supplements. You should divide calcium into 500mg doses throughout the day and consume less than 2000mg of calcium daily. Possible side effects of calcium supplementation are discussed below.

KIDNEY STONES. The most common form of kidney stones contains calcium. Excessive calcium consumption may cause calcium to concentrate in the urinary tract, leading to painful and temporarily disabling stones. Supplemented calcium has been shown to increase the risk of kidney stones more so than dietary calcium.[83]

CARDIOVASCULAR DISEASE. While consuming the recommended daily amount of calcium through **dietary sources** may DECREASE the risk of cardiovascular disease and heart attacks, consuming calcium primarily through **supplements** may actually INCREASE the risk of cardiovascular disease.[84,85] The current recommendation is to obtain at least half of your calcium from dietary sources to minimize this risk.

MALABSORPTION OF IRON AND THYROID HORMONE. If you consume calcium at the same time as iron or thyroid hormone medications, this may decrease your body's ability to absorb these medications. It is recommended that people who take iron or thyroid medication contact their medical provider before starting calcium supplements to discuss proper dosing instructions.

GASTROINTESTINAL COMPLAINTS. Calcium supplements have been associated with gastrointestinal symptoms including upset stomach and constipation. It is best to take calcium with a meal and consume no greater than 500mg at one time to minimize the risk of gastrointestinal side effects.

Why is vitamin D important in osteoporosis care?

Like calcium, vitamin D is essential in maintaining healthy bones. Vitamin D increases the ability of the intestines to absorb calcium and phosphate.[86] In the elderly, it has also been shown to increase muscle strength and decrease fall risk.[87] If you are deficient in vitamin D, your body will only absorb a small fraction of the calcium your consume. As we have previously explored, inadequate calcium levels leads to calcium being pulled from our bones in an effort to maintain blood calcium levels in the proper range. The end result is decreased bone density and increased fracture risk.

What is the difference between vitamin D deficiency and vitamin D insufficiency?

Vitamin D levels are measured using a blood test known as the serum 25-hydroxyvitamin D level. Normal serum 25-hydroxyvitamin D is most commonly reported between 30-50 ng/mL.[88] The distinction between vitamin D deficiency and insufficiency lies in the severity of the condition. Vitamin D **insufficiency** is defined as serum 25-hydroxyvitamin D levels between 21-29 ng/mL and represents a more mild condition. Vitamin D **deficiency** is defined as 25-hydroxyvitamin D levels below 20 ng/mL and represents a more severe condition.

In one study, over 41% of adults have a 25-hydroxyvitamin D level below 20 ng/mL – that means that nearly half of the population is walking around without sufficient vitamin D levels![89]

- **NORMAL VITAMIN D** is defined as serum 25-hydroxyvitamin D between **30-50 ng/mL**
- **VITAMIN D INSUFFICIENCY** is defined as 25-hydroxyvitamin D **21-29 ng/mL**
- **VITAMIN D DEFICIENCY** is defined as serum 25-hydroxyvitamin D **<20 ng/mL**

How much vitamin D should I consume each day?

Vitamin D is unique in that we can obtain our entire recommended daily amount of the vitamin by exposure to sunlight. It has been determined that spending 10 minutes outside in the midday sun during the summer months with exposed arms and legs would produce enough vitamin D for all of our bodily needs. During the winter months, particularly in northern climates, the sun does not produce strong enough ultraviolet rays to meet our vitamin D requirements, and standing outside in a tank top is not exactly practical if you have ever experienced a Minnesota winter!

For the majority of people, **800 IU** of vitamin D is the recommended dose to maintain our vitamin D levels in the normal range. Consuming greater than 4000 IU daily without consulting a medical provider is not recommended as it may increase the risk of side effects. For people with vitamin D deficiency, your medical provider may recommend **50,000 IU of** vitamin D once weekly for 6 to 8 weeks. Once levels return to normal, 800-1000 IU daily should be enough to maintain serum vitamin D levels in the normal range. People with prior gastrointestinal procedures that are unable to maintain vitamin D levels through their diet due to poor absorption of vitamin D may benefit from increased daily doses of vitamin D, or even ultraviolet sunlamps.

How do we obtain vitamin D?

Vitamin D is primarily obtained through sunlight exposure and oral supplements. Food sources may contain vitamin D, but most would find it difficult to obtain the necessary amount of vitamin D from food sources alone. Below is a list of common sources of vitamin D.

SUNLIGHT EXPOSURE (ULTRAVIOLET B RAYS). Sunlight exposure, particularly exposure to the UVB rays, is the most common source of vitamin D. The UVB rays are absorbed by the skin and, through a series of steps, are converted into vitamin D. A number of factors can negatively impact our body's ability to convert UVB into vitamin D. For instance, darkly pigmented skin, advancing age, and use of certain medications will decrease vitamin D production in the body. In addition, the sun's UVB rays simply are not strong enough in northern climates to produce vitamin D throughout the majority of winter months. During those times, the body relies completely on dietary sources of vitamin D.

COMMERCIALLY FORTIFIED MILK. Milk is often fortified with small amounts of vitamin D – typically 100 IU per 8-ounce glass. Between the calcium and the vitamin D content, a glass of milk really does do a body good!

COD LIVER OIL. Cod liver oil is an excellent source of vitamin D. It can be taken by the tablespoon for the adventurous folks, but is also available in capsule form.

MUSHROOMS EXPOSED TO SUNLIGHT. Mushrooms, including portabella and maitake that have been exposed to ultraviolet light, can contain upwards of 400-900 IU of vitamin D.

VITAMIN D SUPPLEMENTATION. Oral vitamin D supplements are an economical and taste bud friendly way to reach your daily vitamin D requirements!

Should I supplement with vitamin D2 or vitamin D3?

If you walk down the aisles of your local pharmacy, you may find that vitamin D comes in two forms – vitamin D3 (cholecalciferol) and vitamin D2 (ergocalciferol). In general, both forms have a similar effect on blood vitamin D levels and either is perfectly acceptable as a dietary supplement for vitamin D.[90] Some studies have suggested that vitamin D3 may have a greater impact on blood vitamin D levels compared to vitamin D2. From my personal experience with patients, I have not seen a significant difference between the two forms of vitamin D. Both appear relatively equal in their ability to raise serum 25-hydroxyvitamin D levels and I would consider them equally effective supplements.

What are possible side effects of vitamin D supplementation?

As with all medications and supplements, too much of a good thing can lead to side effects. In regard to vitamin D, excessive supplementation – especially when combined with high levels of calcium, can lead to high blood calcium levels (hypercalcemia), high urine calcium levels (hypercalciuria), and increased risk of developing kidney stones.[88] Chronically high levels of vitamin D outside of the normal range has also been linked to the increased risk of pancreatic cancer, prostate cancer, and increased mortality.[91,92] Please consult your medical provider before considering those mega-doses of vitamin D that you may have read about!

How does calcium and vitamin D supplementation affect bone mineral density and fracture risk?

Hopefully it is apparent by now that calcium is critically important in building healthy, mineralized bones and that vitamin D helps the body absorb calcium. If we are deficient in either, it can lead to worsening bone health and progression of osteoporosis… but does supplementation of calcium and vitamin D alone increase bone density AND decrease the risk of sustaining a fracture? A large study spanning 7 years involving 36,282 postmenopausal women aimed to answer this question. Women between the ages of 50 and 79 were given 1000 mg of calcium and 400 IU of vitamin D daily or were provided with a placebo. The results are discussed below.

BONE DENSITY. Both groups of patients, including those receiving calcium and vitamin D supplements as well as those receiving the placebo, experienced a DECREASE in the bone density at the hip over the 7 year duration of the study. However, patients taking calcium and vitamin D lost 1.06% less hip bone density than those receiving the placebo, which was the only significant result of the study. Interestingly, bone density actually INCREASED by 2-3% at the spine in both groups of patients, but these results were not significant because both the patients taking the supplements, as well as the patients receiving the placebo experienced this same increase in bone density! **The researchers provided an accurate overview of the effect of calcium and vitamin D supplementation in this article. However, you can see how it would be easy for a secondary author reviewing the article to claim that calcium and vitamin D supplementation can increase bone density by 3%, which it did at the spine! But those results are meaningless because this secondary author would have conveniently left out that patients taking a placebo also improved their bone density by the same amount!**

FRACTURE RISK. Calcium and vitamin D supplementation has not been shown to reduce the risk of sustaining hip or spine fractures. Women receiving the calcium and vitamin D supplements did have 12% less hip fractures throughout the course of the study compared to the placebo group, however, this was not considered statistically significant. This means that while a difference was observed, the change was not great enough to say whether the supplements actually decreased the risk of fracture, or whether the difference occurred purely by chance.

RESULTS AT A GLANCE	
DOES CALCIUM AND VITAMIN D IMPROVE BONE DENSITY?	At the hip, patients taking calcium and vitamin D supplements lost 1.06% less bone density over time compared to placebo. At the spine, these supplements did not impact bone density compared to placebo.
DOES CALCIUM AND VITAMIN D DECREASE FRACTURE RISK?	There was a 12% decrease in hip fractures in patients taking calcium and vitamin D, however, these results were not found to be significant by the researchers.

The overall conclusion by the authors of this large, well designed study was that supplementation led to a small improvement in bone density at the hip and may slow the progression of osteoporosis. However, calcium and vitamin D did not prevent fractures. Calcium and vitamin D are important adjuncts in maintaining bone health, but should not be the sole treatment in managing osteoporosis.

Key Points

- Calcium is an important building block for the structural integrity of bone.
- Vitamin D is necessary for the body to absorb dietary calcium in our intestines.
- If the dietary intake of calcium and vitamin D cannot maintain blood calcium levels within the normal range, the body will pull calcium from the bones to maintain these levels – at the expense of bone density!
- The recommended daily calcium dose is 1200 mg. Ideally, at least half of your daily calcium should come from dietary sources.
- The recommended daily vitamin D dose is 800-1000 IU. This may be obtained through sunlight exposure, dietary sources, or supplementation.
- Calcium and vitamin D supplementation has been shown to slow the loss of hip bone density compared to placebo.
- Calcium and vitamin D supplementation has not been shown to have a significant impact on reducing the risk of hip or spine fractures.

- It is best to consult your medical provider before you begin taking any new vitamin supplements.

10 | Estrogen

GENERIC NAME	ESTRADIOL
BRAND NAME	ESTRACE, PREMARIN, ESTRADERM, VIVELLE
ROUTE	ORAL PILLS, TRANSDERMAL PATCHES
DOSE	LOWEST EFFECTIVE DOSE (VARIES)

How does estrogen treat osteoporosis?

Estrogens are widely prescribed for the purposes of birth control, management of those terrible menopausal symptoms (including the dreaded hot flashes!), as well as the prevention and management of osteoporosis in select women. The theory behind prescribing this class of medications in postmenopausal women who are at risk of developing osteoporosis is logical. The abrupt loss of estrogen during menopause leads to a profound decrease in bone density – often greater than 10% of bone is lost in just a few short years! Supplementing estrogen reverses this hormonal imbalance. Estrogens have been shown to increase the activity of osteoblasts (bone-building cells) and decrease the activity of osteoclasts (bone-recycling cells).[94] Estrogen improves muscular strength and balance, which decreases the risk of falls and associated fractures.[95-97] In our intestines, estrogen works to increase calcium absorption.[98] As you can see, estrogen has a positive influence on our bone health.

How effective is estrogen at treating osteoporosis?

When evaluating any treatment for osteoporosis, we must critically evaluate whether the medication improves bone density AND decreases the risk of sustaining a fracture. Let's review some of the pertinent studies evaluating the effectiveness of estrogen in the management of osteoporosis.

BONE DENSITY. A meta-analysis of 57 studies between 1966 and 1999 was performed by a group of researchers to determine the effect of estrogen on bone density.[99] These studies compared postmenopausal women who received estrogen to those receiving a placebo – either an inactive medication or a combination of calcium and vitamin D without estrogen. The women in the studies had DXA bone density scans prior to starting treatment and again at least 1 year afterwards. When compared to patients receiving the placebo, the women taking estrogen experienced on average an increase of **5.4% in spine bone density, 2.5% in hip bone density, and 3.0% in wrist bone density**.

FRACTURE RISK. The Women's Health Initiative Study began in the late 1990s and sought to determine if estrogen supplementation decreases the risk of sustaining a fragility fracture.[100] Over 16,000 postmenopausal women between the ages of 50 and 79 received either estrogen only, estrogen with an added progestin (for endometrial protection in women with a uterus) or a placebo. The results were impressive – estrogen and estrogen with an added progestin **decreased the risk of sustaining a spine fracture by 36%, hip fracture by 35%, and all other fractures by 29%** compared to placebo. The trial was planned for 8.5 years, but the estrogen with progestin group of patients were stopped from continuing after an average of 5.2 years once it was determined that negative health outcomes were occurring as a result of taking the medication. These included increased risk of heart attack, stroke, pulmonary embolism (a blood clot in the lungs), and invasive breast cancer. It should be known that patients in the trial received a relatively high dose of oral estrogen with progestin. More recent studies have suggested that transdermal (skin) patches and lower doses of estrogen medications may be associated with fewer side effects. Estrogen is clearly effective at reducing the risk of fractures, but both the risks and benefits estrogen must be carefully considered.

RESULTS AT A GLANCE	
DOES ESTROGEN IMPROVE BONE DENSITY?	Patients taking estrogen experienced a 5.4% increase in spine bone density, 2.5% increase in hip bone density, and 3.0% increase in wrist bone density.
DOES ESTROGEN DECREASE FRACTURE RISK?	Patients taking estrogen had a 36% decreased risk of spine fracture, 35% decreased risk of hip fracture, and 29% decreased risk of all other

What are the adverse effects of estrogen?

Your medical provider must carefully balance the benefits of estrogen with the risks associated with use of this medication. Many people falsely associate hormonal treatments as being completely "natural" and "safe." That is not necessarily the case for all patients. Below is a list of possible side effects associated with the use of estrogens in postmenopausal women.

BREAST AND ENDOMETRIAL CANCER. Approximately two-thirds of breast and endometrial (the inner lining of the uterus) cancer are estrogen receptor positive – meaning when estrogen binds to the tumor it acts as fuel to stimulate its growth. The risk of developing these forms of cancer is associated with the number of years a patient is exposed to estrogen. A patient who experiences early menopause (before age 50) and supplements estrogen for a period of time does not experience an increased risk of breast and endometrial cancer.[101] However, postmenopausal women age 50 and older who supplement estrogen for 5 or more years have an increased lifetime risk of developing breast and endometrial cancer.[101-103]

THROMBOEMBOLIC DISEASE. Women who take estrogen are at increased risk of developing blood clots.[104] Blood clots will typically present themselves as a **deep venous thrombosis** – or a stationary blood clot in the deep veins of the legs. This is managed with blood thinning medications and activity modification until the clot resolves. An **embolism** refers to a blood clot which has broken off and become mobile. These can lodge in the lungs, where they are known as a pulmonary embolism. This is a potentially life threatening medical condition that requires emergency medical intervention.

GALLBLADDER DISEASE. Women taking estrogen are at increased risk for developing stones in the gallbladder called gallstones (more technically known as cholelithiasis). If these stones remain stationary in the gallbladder, then it is unlikely that they will cause any symptoms. However, if a large gallstone exits into the tube that connects the gallbladder to the intestines it may become stuck – causing significant pain, inflammation, fever, and vomiting. This medical condition, known as cholecystitis (inflammation of the gallbladder) may even require surgical treatment. [105]

STROKE. There is an increased risk of stroke in people taking oral estrogen, which appears to be related to dose and duration of treatment with estrogen.[106]

What dose of estrogen is necessary to treat osteoporosis?

In 2004, a group of researchers evaluated data from the Million Women Study to determine how different doses and routes of administration (pills vs. skin patches) of estrogen only and estrogen with progestin affected fracture risk.[107] A total of 138,737 postmenopausal women between the ages of 50 and 69 were included in the study. Women with a prior hysterectomy were given oral or skin patches with estrogen only, whereas patients with a uterus were given estrogen with an added progestin at varying doses. Patients were followed for up to 4 years to determine the reduction in fracture risk. **Overall, all routes of administration, doses, and forms of hormonal therapy did not vary significantly in their ability to reduce fractures**. The researchers concluded that lower doses of hormonal therapy (oral estradiol less than 1 mg, oral equine estrogen less than 0.625 mg, transdermal estradiol <50 ug) appeared to be as effective at reducing fracture risk as higher doses of these medications and were associated with fewer side effects.

Once I stop taking estrogen, what happens to my bone density and fracture risk?

It has been well established that estrogen is effective at increasing bone density and decreasing fracture risk while the patient is taking the medication. But are these effects long-lived after a patient stops taking the medication? Reviewing the available research, it appears that the bone protective effects of estrogen are short lived. Patients experience a rapid decline in bone density and increase in fracture risk similar to if they had never taken estrogen within 1 to 2 years of stopping the medication.[107] If you stop taking hormone therapy for osteoporosis, it is recommended that you are transitioned to another osteoporosis medication to maintain your improved bone density and decreased fracture risk.

The bottom line on using estrogen to treat osteoporosis...

Women experience an abrupt loss of estrogen production associated with decreased bone density and increased fracture risk following menopause. It seems natural that supplementing estrogen would improve bone density and decrease the risk of sustaining a fracture, and it does! However, this is not without side effects which must be carefully considered. No consensus in the medical community currently exists regarding the use of hormone replacement therapy in the prevention and treatment of postmenopausal osteoporosis. Estrogen can be considered for postmenopausal women who are younger than 60 years old with osteoporosis. In women with a uterus (no prior hysterectomy), a progestin should be added to the estrogen for endometrial protection. Given the potential side effects, it is best to avoid estrogens in women over 60 years old and in patients with a history of breast cancer, endometrial cancer, blood clots, heart disease, or uncontrolled hypertension (high blood pressure). In select patients, estrogen is an excellent option for managing osteoporosis that is associated with menopause.

11   The Bisphonates

GENERIC NAME	ALENDRONATE
BRAND NAME	FOSAMAX
ROUTE	ORAL PILLS
DOSE	10 MG DAILY OR 70 MG WEEKLY

GENERIC NAME	RISEDRONATE
BRAND NAME	ACTONEL
ROUTE	ORAL PILLS
DOSE	5 MG DAILY, 35 MG WEEKLY, OR 150 MG MONTHLY

GENERIC NAME	ZOLEDRONIC ACID
BRAND NAME	RECLAST
ROUTE	INTRAVENOUS INFUSION PERFORMED BY A MEDICAL PROFESSIONAL
DOSE	5 MG YEARLY

How do bisphonates treat osteoporosis?

Bisphonates were the first class of medications developed for the treatment of osteoporosis. Since these medications have been available for so long, there have been countless studies proving that bisphonates effectively increase bone density and decrease fracture risk. Bisphonates have also been used to treat hypercalcemia (high levels of calcium in the blood), Paget's disease, and as an adjunct in certain cancers (multiple myeloma, prostate and breast cancers) to decrease the risk of fracture. Bisphonates are available in both oral and IV forms.

How exactly do bisphonates work? The process is fairly complicated, but if we break it down into the a few key steps it becomes much easier to understand.

- **STEP 1.** Bisphosphonates are absorbed into our bloodstream. Intravenous bisphosphonates enter directly into our bloodstream, whereas the pill form must be absorbed in our intestines. Dosing instructions for the pill form of bisphosphonates should be carefully followed because only 1% of the medication is actually absorbed into our bloodstreams! [108]
- **STEP 2.** Bisphosphonates travel through our bloodstream until they reach our bones. Here, they attach to locations where osteoclasts had previously recycled old bone. [109]
- **STEP 3.** Bisphosphonates enter into the osteoclast cells, and once inside, bisphosphonates inhibit important enzymes necessary for osteoclasts to continue recycling old bone. [110,111] This shuts down the speed at which osteoclast cells work. [112] Osteoblast (bone building) cell activity is also slowed, but less significantly than osteoclasts, allowing for improved bone density and decreased risk of fractures! [113,114]

Have you ever heard of a "drug holiday" when discussing osteoporosis with your medical provider? It may sound like sipping on a margarita while swinging in a hammock… and that really isn't too far off. It is a concept that applies only to bisphosphonates due to a unique feature of these medications. Most treatments that improve bone health stop working when you stop taking them – but bisphosphonates can continue to protect your bones for many years! This is important because it allows patients to completely stop taking osteoporosis medications for a period of time while maintaining their bone health. As long as your risk of sustaining a fracture in the near future isn't high, studies have shown that those taking Fosamax and Actonel for 5 years may stop the medication for up to 5 years with periodic monitoring. Similarly, patients taking Reclast for 3 years may consider a 3 year drug holiday. For patients who are not interested in taking medications for long periods of time, drug holidays are a welcomed concept.

How effective are bisphosphonates at treating osteoporosis?

When evaluating any treatment for osteoporosis, we must critically evaluate whether the medication improves bone density and decreases the risk of sustaining a fracture. Let's review some of the pertinent studies evaluating the effectiveness of each of the bisphosphonates in the management of osteoporosis.

FOSAMAX: BONE DENSITY AND FRACTURE RISK. Fosamax is one of the oldest, and therefore, one of the most studied oral medications developed for the treatment of osteoporosis. Over the years, several studies with thousands of patients have proven the effectiveness and relative safety of Fosamax. One such study known as The Fracture Intervention Trial (FIT) began in the early 1990s. The results of this study led to Fosamax being the first FDA approved medication for treatment of osteoporosis. The effects of Fosamax in two separate groups of patients were evaluated – those with a prior fragility fracture (spine fracture) and those with a diagnosis of osteoporosis (hip T-score less than -2.5). The results will be discussed below.

The first subset of the trial consisted of 2027 postmenopausal women between the ages of 55 and 81 **with a prior spine fracture.**[115] Patients received either Fosamax or a placebo (calcium 1000 mg and vitamin D 250 IU daily) for 3 years. Patients receiving Fosamax had a bone density increase of 6.2% at the spine and 4.1% at the hip. This led to a 50% and 30% reduced risk of fracture respectively at these locations!

The second subset of the trial consisted of 4432 postmenopausal women between the ages 51 and 84 **without a prior spine fracture, but with a hip T-score less than -2.5.**[116] Once again, patients received either Fosamax or a placebo for 4 years. Patients receiving Fosamax had a bone density increase of 8.3% at the spine and 3.8% at the hip. Interestingly, patients taking the calcium and vitamin D placebo experienced a bone density increase of 1.5% at the spine, but a loss of 0.8% at the hip. Compared to patients receiving the placebo, Fosamax decreased the risk of sustaining a hip fracture by 56% and a spine fracture by 44%!

ACTONEL: BONE DENSITY AND FRACTURE RISK. Similar to Fosamax, Actonel is an oral medication used to manage osteoporosis. The Vertebral Efficacy with Risedronate (VERT) trial compared the effectiveness of Actonel in two subsets of patients.[117] The first included 2458 postmenopausal women with **one prior spine fracture and a spine T-score <-2.0** compared to a placebo (1000 mg calcium and 500 IU vitamin D). Over a 3 year period, patients taking Actonel experienced a bone density increase of 5.4% at the spine and 1.6% at the hip. This was associated with a decreased spine fracture risk of 41% and a decreased hip fracture risk of 39%! In the second subset of patients, 1226 postmenopausal women with **two or more prior spine fractures** received either Actonel or a placebo for three years. Use of Actonel led to a 49% decreased risk of spine fracture and 33% decreased risk of hip fracture compared to the placebo group in patients with multiple prior fragility fractures!

RECLAST: BONE DENSITY AND FRACTURE RISK. Reclast treats osteoporosis the same way as Fosamax and Actonel, however, Reclast is administered via once yearly IV infusions instead of pills. The Health Outcomes and Reduced Incidence with Zoledronic Acid Once Yearly (HORIZON) trial aimed to determine the effects of Reclast on bone density and fracture risk.[118] A total of 7765 postmenopausal women were selected for the trial. Eligible patients had a **hip T-score less than -2.5 or a T-score less than -1.5 with x-ray evidence of 2 prior spine fractures**. After the completion of the 3 year study, patients receiving Reclast had a bone density increase of 6.71% at the spine and 5.06% at the hip. This was associated with a remarkable 70% decreased risk of spine fracture and 41% decreased risk of hip fracture compared to placebo!

RESULTS AT A GLANCE	
DO BISPHOSPHONATES IMPROVE BONE DENSITY?	Patients taking bisphosphonates experienced a 5.4% to 8.5% increase in spine bone density, and a 1.6% to 5.06% increase in hip bone density.
DO BISPHOSPHONATES DECREASE FRACTURE RISK?	Patients taking bisphosphonates had a 44% to 70% decreased risk of spine fracture, and a 30% to 56% decreased risk of hip fracture.

What are the adverse effects of bisphosphonates?

Your medical provider must balance the benefits of bisphosphonates with the risks associated with use of these medications. Several large studies have reported no significant difference in adverse symptoms when comparing the group of patients taking bisphosphonates to those taking a placebo if the medications are taken appropriately.[115-117] However, failure to follow dosing instructions and long term use of these medications has been associated with certain adverse events which must be carefully considered. Below is a list of possible side effects associated with the use of bisphosphonates.

ATYPICAL FEMUR FRACTURES. You might think that any fracture of the femur is "atypical," and you are correct! In the orthopedic world, however, we know that bones tend to break in predictable locations and patterns. When bones break in a location that we wouldn't expect, we say it is atypical. Atypical fractures of the hip refer to a stress fractures that are not located by the ball and socket joint of the hip, but along the shaft of the bone in the middle and upper thigh region. It is quite rare in patients taking bisphosphonates and no studies have definitively shown that bisphosphonates actually *cause* atypical femur fractures. However, there has been an increased incidence noted in patients taking bisphosphonates, especially in patients taking this class of medications longer than 5-10 years. This is an important consideration, particularly in younger patients with osteoporosis that may require long-term treatment to decrease the risk of fractures over many years or even decades. When an atypical femur fracture develops, patients often report a slow onset of pain in the thigh that gradually worsens and can progress to a complete fracture if not treated appropriately.[119] To show how rare this complication is, consider the following statistic– several large studies including over 10,000 patients taking Fosamax for 10+ years have failed to report a single case of an atypical femur fracture.[115,116,118] The bottom line is that bisphosphonates prevent far more fractures than they cause. Discuss this possible side effect with your medical provider to learn the facts.

OSTEONECROSIS OF THE JAW (ONJ). Osteonecrosis of the jaw is defined as exposed jaw bone that does not heal within 8 weeks.[120] This has been reported as a possible side effect in patients taking bisphosphonates for extended periods of time, particularly those with poor oral hygiene, those requiring dental extraction surgeries, and in patients with cancer taking chemotherapy. As with atypical femur fractures, no studies have definitively shown bisphosphonates to *cause* ONJ, but it has been reported to occur at a greater rate in patients taking bisphosphonates compared to the general population. This side effect is extremely rare – with less than 1 case reported per 100,000 patient years of treatment. In the FLEX trial, there were no reported cases of ONJ, even in patients taking Fosamax for 10 years.[121] In the HORIZON study, there was 1 reported case of ONJ in a patient taking Reclast, as well as 1 reported case in the placebo group – indicating that this condition can occur in the general population as well. Carefully consider this side effect if you have a history of gum disease or if you anticipate the need for significant dental work while taking bisphosphonates.

GASTROINTESTINAL DISEASE. Gastrointestinal disease refers to common conditions including acid reflux, inflammation of the esophagus (the tube connecting the mouth to the stomach) and even ulceration of the esophagus and stomach. When taken properly, with a full glass of water on an empty stomach followed by sitting upright for at least 30 minutes, oral bisphosphonates have not been shown to increase the risk of gastrointestinal disease when compared to patients taking a placebo. If taken inappropriately, bisphosphonates can increase the risk of gastrointestinal disease. It is even safe to take bisphosphonates if you have a history of acid reflux and stomach ulcers. If you have a medical condition that makes it more likely to have food or pills get stuck in the throat or esophagus, it is best to avoid the pill form of these medications to avoid risking injury to the esophagus.

ESOPHAGEAL CANCER. An older study out of the United Kingdom indicated that use of bisphosphonates longer than 5 years was associated with an increased risk of esophageal cancer.[122] In this study, it was estimated that 1 in 1000 people in the general population will be diagnosed with esophageal cancer, while the rate in patients taking bisphosphonates was 2 in 1000. More recent research has failed to link bisphosphonate use of any duration to esophageal cancer.[123] Despite these more recent findings, patients with an increased risk of esophageal cancer should discuss this risk factor with their medical provider to determine if oral bisphosphonates are the best treatment option to manage their osteoporosis.

FLU-LIKE SYMPTOMS. Flu-like symptoms are commonly experienced by patients who receive an IV infusion of Reclast. With the first infusion, these symptoms can be expected in as many as 32% of patients.[124] Symptoms begin 24-36 hours after the dose is given and can last for 3 days. Luckily, this is uncommon with future infusions on years 2 and 3, when only 2.8% to 6.6% of patients report these symptoms. To minimize the risk of developing these symptoms, patients are encouraged to take acetaminophen (Tylenol) for 1-2 days prior and for 3 days following Reclast. Tylenol has been shown to decrease the odds of developing these symptoms by 50% or greater.

HYPOCALCEMIA. Transient hypocalcemia, or a temporary drop in blood calcium levels, has been reported in certain patients taking bisphosphonates.[125] Patients that develop symptoms from hypocalcemia generally have an underlying medical condition which makes them susceptible to the condition – including low levels of vitamin D or certain forms of cancer. Your medical provider should ensure that blood calcium and vitamin D levels are normal prior to starting this class of medications, and if you are at increased risk of developing hypocalcemia, it may be recommended to have your calcium levels monitored periodically.

KIDNEY DISEASE. Kidney disease, including kidney failure, has been reported in certain patients taking bisphosphonates.[126] While rare, patients at risk of developing kidney disease include those with a history of underlying kidney disease or multiple myeloma, as well as in patients who take diuretics or long term nonsteroidal anti-inflammatory medications. The general recommendation is to avoid bisphosphonates if you have stage 4 or stage 5 kidney disease.

HEART ARRHYTHMIA. Transient heart arrhythmias, or a temporarily abnormal heartbeat, have been reported in patients taking bisphosphonates.[127] In the HORIZON trial, 6.9% of patients taking Reclast experienced a heart arrhythmia compared to 5.3% of the placebo patients. In the trial, there were no reported adverse events from these temporary arrhythmias such as heart attack or stroke.

MUSCULOSKELETAL PAIN. Muscle and joint pain is a common reported adverse event in patients taking bisphosphonates. In rare cases, severe muscle pain has developed in patients; prompting a switch to another osteoporosis medication.

What dose of bisphosphonates is necessary to treat osteoporosis?

Fosamax is available in oral pills and can be taken 10mg daily, or more commonly, 70mg once weekly. Actonel is also available in oral pills and can be taken as 5mg daily, 35mg weekly, or 150mg monthly. Coated tablets that are easier on the stomach are also available for Actonel. Reclast is only available in IV form and is administered once yearly as a 5mg dose.

Once I stop taking bisphosphonates, what happens to my bone density and fracture risk?

Bisphosphonate medications are unique in that their bone protective effects last for several years after you stop taking them. If a patient wishes to stop taking other osteoporosis medications including estrogens, Prolia, or Forteo, they must transition to another medication to "lock in" the increased bone density or jeopardize losing the benefits of these medications rapidly over a period of 1 or 2 years. With bisphosphonates, this is not the case. Separate studies have examined what happens to bone density and fracture risk once a patient stops taking each of the bisphosphonates... so let's see what happens!

The Fracture Intervention Long-Term Extension Trial (FLEX) consisted of 1099 postmenopausal women from the FIT study who had previously taken 5 years of Fosamax.[121] The patients were given either an additional 5 years of Fosamax (10 years total) or were switched to a placebo (500 mg calcium and 250 IU vitamin D) for that time. In regard to bone density, patients who transitioned into the placebo group did experience a very slow decrease in bone density compared to those who remained on Fosamax for the full 10 years. However, despite this small drop in bone density, the majority of placebo patients continued to have ongoing bone protection from their initial 5 years of Fosamax! **Patients receiving 5 years of Fosamax followed by 5 years of a placebo had the same reduced fracture risk as patients receiving the full 10 years of Fosamax!** The only exception was patients who were high risk for ongoing fracture, including those with a T-score remaining below -2.5 after 5 years of treatment, and those that have had a prior painful spine fracture. For these high risk patients, it is best to continue Fosamax for a total of 10 years as the bone protective effects were not found to be as long lasting.

The VERT Extension Study included 759 postmenopausal women from the original VERT trial who had previously received 3 years of Actonel.[128] Following a one year drug holiday, patients experienced a decrease in spine and hip bone mineral density of 0.83% and 1.23% respectively compared to their bone mass after 3 years of Actonel. Despite this decrease, bone density remained higher when compared to patients who had never received Actonel. Interestingly, **patients who had been given 3 years of Actonel followed by a 1 year drug holiday still had a 46% decrease risk of sustaining a new spine fracture compared to patients who never received Actonel** – indicating the bone protective effects of this medication last at least 1 year after the patient stops taking it. The general recommendation is to treat Fosamax and Actonel the same in relation to drug holidays – patients with a low risk of fracture following 5 years of treatment are eligible for a 5 year drug holiday.

The HORIZON Extension Study included 1233 postmenopausal women from the original HORIZON trial.[129] All patients had previously received 3 years of Reclast. Patients were divided into two groups – those that would receive an additional 3 years of Reclast (6 years total), or those that would receive 3 years of a placebo. At the end of the trial, patients who received an additional 3 years of Reclast experienced an additional bone density increase of 0.24% at the spine and 3.2% at the hip. Patients receiving the placebo had a decrease of 0.80% at the spine, but an increase of 1.18% at the hip. **There was no significant difference in the rate of**

new fractures between those receiving 6 years of Reclast and those who had 3 years of the medication followed by 3 years of the placebo. These findings indicate that a 3 year drug holiday should be considered in all patients after 3 years of Reclast.

The bottom line on using bisphosphonates to treat osteoporosis...

Bisphosphonates are the oldest class of osteoporosis medications which has allowed us to collect years of scientific research proving their relative safety and effectiveness. They work by decreasing the number and activity of osteoclasts – allowing the bone building osteoblasts to catch up and increase our bone density! Long term studies of both oral and IV forms have shown that they decrease the risk of fracture by 50% or greater! Bisphosphonates are unique in that their bone protective effects have been shown to last for 3-5 years after stopping the medication entirely – allowing for a period in which you do not need to take any medication, known as a drug holiday. However, there are important possible side effects to consider. Use of bisphosphonates longer than 5 years increases the risk of sustaining an atypical femur fracture or developing osteonecrosis of the jaw, though these are very rare side effects. Patients should monitor for abnormal thigh and jaw pain and report these symptoms immediately to their medical provider if they develop. When taken appropriately, bisphosphonates have not been shown to increase the risk of gastrointestinal irritation or esophageal cancer even in patients with pre-existing acid reflux disease. It is best to avoid bisphosphonates in patients with severe renal disease and patients on dialysis. Bisphosphonates were the first medication specifically designed for managing osteoporosis, and they remain an important option for those wishing to improve their bone health.

12 | Denosumab (Prolia)

GENERIC NAME	DENOSUMAB
BRAND NAME	PROLIA
ROUTE	INJECTION INTO THE SUBCUTANEOUS SKIN TISSUE PERFORMED BY A MEDICAL PROFESSIONAL
DOSE	60 MG EVERY 6 MONTHS

How does Prolia treat osteoporosis?

To understand how Prolia is used to manage osteoporosis, one must understand the RANK-RANKL-OPG Pathway which was discussed in the first section of this text. To review, the bone building cells (osteoblasts) and building recycling cells (osteoclasts) communicate with one another to ensure that the rate of old bone being recycled and the rate of new bone being created are equal. The osteoblasts are the generals who lead the way – these cells release a molecule called **RANKL** which acts as an "ON" signal for the osteoclast cells to begin breaking down old bone. Osteoblasts also release a molecule called **OPG** which acts as an "OFF" signal for osteoclasts to stop breaking down old bone to allow the osteoblast cells to fill in the region with new, healthy bone.[130] **An imbalance between the rate of old bone being broken down and new bone being created can lead to a loss of bone mass over time and ultimately, osteoporosis.** But what if a medication were created to control these signals? This is where Prolia makes its dramatic entrance!

Prolia is a medication used to treat osteoporosis, as well as hypercalcemia of malignancy (elevated blood calcium levels due to certain types of cancer).[131] Prolia is an antibody which binds RANKL. In doing so, Prolia shuts down this line of communication between osteoblasts and osteoclasts, leading to decreased bone breakdown and a chance for the bone-building osteoblast cells to "catch up" in laying new bone. This medication has been shown in clinical studies to increase bone density, increase the thickness of cortical bone, and decrease the risk of sustaining a fragility fracture.[132]

How effective is Prolia at treating osteoporosis?

When evaluating any treatment for osteoporosis, we must critically evaluate whether the medication improves bone density and decreases the risk of sustaining a fracture. Let's review some of the pertinent studies evaluating the effectiveness of Prolia in the management of osteoporosis.

BONE DENSITY IN POSTMENOPAUSAL WOMEN. A number of scientific studies have been performed to determine the effectiveness of Prolia in improving bone density in postmenopausal women. The FREEDOM trial was a 3 year study that included 4550 postmenopausal women between the ages of 60 and 90 with confirmed osteoporosis.[133] The placebo group was given at least 1000 mg of calcium and 400 IU of vitamin D daily for comparison. **At the conclusion of the 3 year trial, patients treated with Prolia experienced a bone density increase of 9.2% at the spine and 6% at the hip** compared to 0% at both locations for the placebo patients. The trial was extended for an additional 3 years (6 years total) in the FREEDOM extension trial. **Patients receiving 6 years of Prolia experienced a total bone mineral density increase of 15.2% at the spine and 7.5% at the hip!** Other studies spanning 8 years have reported bone density increases of 16.5% at the spine and 6.8% at the hip.[134]

BONE DENSITY IN MEN. The ADAMO trial sought to determine the effectiveness of Prolia in men (a group that is often neglected in most osteoporosis studies!).[135] The study included 242 men with low bone density or a prior fragility fracture. Men received either Prolia for 2 years or a placebo, which consisted of at least 1000 mg of calcium and 800 IU of vitamin D daily. **Men receiving 2 years of Prolia experienced a bone density increase of 5.7% at the spine and 2.4% at the hip**, compared to the placebo group which experienced little to no change at either location. There was no statistically significant difference in side effects between men treated with Prolia and those who received the placebo.

FRACTURE RISK. The Pivotal Fracture Study included 7808 postmenopausal women with osteoporosis between the ages of 60-91.[133] Patients in the trial received 3 years of Prolia compared to the placebo group, which consisted of calcium and vitamin D supplementation. The primary goal of the study was to determine if Prolia decreased the risk of sustaining fragility fractures. **After 3 years, patients receiving Prolia had a 68% reduced risk of spine fracture, 40% reduced risk of hip fracture, and 20% reduced risk of all other fractures** compared to patients receiving the placebo!

RESULTS AT A GLANCE	
DOES PROLIA IMPROVE BONE DENSITY?	Patients taking Prolia experienced a 5.7% to 16.5% increase in spine bone density, and a 2.4% to 7.5% increase in hip bone density following 2 to 8 years of treatment.
DOES PROLIA DECREASE FRACTURE RISK?	Patients taking Prolia had a 68% decreased risk of spine fracture, and a 40% decreased risk of hip fracture following 3 years of treatment.

What are the adverse effects of Prolia?

Your medical provider must balance the benefits of the Prolia with the risks associated with use of this medication. Studies spanning 8 years have indicated Prolia to be a safe and effective medication, however, below is a list of potential side effects which must be carefully considered.

HYPOCALCEMIA. Transient hypocalcemia, or a temporary drop in blood calcium levels, has been reported in patients taking Prolia.[197] The risk is greatest in patients with hypoparathyroidism, chronic kidney disease, and gastrointestinal disorders which cause malabsorption of vitamins and minerals. Hypocalcemia often produces no symptoms before blood calcium levels return to normal, but there have been a few reported cases of severe symptoms in patients with end stage renal failure who are on dialysis. Your medical provider will assess your calcium levels prior to starting Prolia and if you are at risk of developing hypocalcemia, a second lab test measuring your blood calcium levels may be performed 10-14 days after starting the medication. It is important for you to consume enough calcium daily to maintain blood calcium levels in the normal range while taking this medication.

OSTEONECROSIS OF THE JAW. Osteonecrosis of the jaw is defined as exposed jaw bone that does not heal within 8 weeks. This has been reported as a possible side effect in patients taking Prolia for extended periods of time, particularly patients with poor oral hygiene, those requiring dental extraction surgeries, and in patients with cancer taking chemotherapy. In the FREEDOM extension trial, 6 patients out of 4550 developed osteonecrosis of the jaw over a 6 year period. A separate study monitoring the effects of Prolia over an 8 year period reported no cases of this condition. As with the bisphosphonates, it is important to maintain good oral hygiene and have routine dental examinations while taking Prolia to minimize the risk of this side effect.

ATYPICAL FEMUR FRACTURES. Atypical femur fractures include fractures of the shaft portion of the femur bone as opposed to the ball and socket region of the hip. These fractures often cause symptoms including a nagging thigh pain for days or weeks prior to fracturing. The cause and effect relationship between Prolia and atypical femur fractures has not been clearly established, but patients taking Prolia have experienced these types of fractures. In the FREEDOM extension trial, 1 patient out of 4550 experienced an atypical femur fracture over the 6 year duration of the trial. A separate study monitoring the effects of Prolia over an 8 year period reported no cases of atypical femur fractures. While rare, you should watch for abnormal thigh pain and report this symptom immediately to your medical provider in order to receive appropriate treatment to minimize the risk of fracturing.

IMMUNE SYSTEM. The immune system is our defense against infections. The RANKL that Prolia blocks has also been shown to have a role in certain aspects of the immune system.[136] Studies have indicated that patients taking Prolia are at increased risk of developing infections that require hospitalization.[137] This risk is greatest in patients with compromised immune systems due to medical conditions or use of medications which weaken the immune system. Patients taking Prolia should closely watch for signs and symptoms of infection and report these immediately to their medical provider.

MUSCULOSKELETAL PAIN. Pain in the muscles and joints is the most commonly reported side effect of Prolia. These symptoms are typically mild and temporary, but occasionally are more severe – leading patients to switch to other osteoporosis medications.

What dose of Prolia is necessary to treat osteoporosis?

Prolia is administered by injection into the subcutaneous tissue of the skin by a medical professional every 6 months. The FDA approved dose of Prolia is 60mg.

Once I stop taking Prolia, what happens to my bone density and fracture risk?

Prolia has been proven to increase bone density and decrease fracture risk, however, these effects are short-lived after you stop taking the medication. One study provided osteoporotic postmenopausal women 2 years of Prolia followed by no treatment for the next 2 years.[138] After 2 years without treatment, bone density decreased by 6.6% at the spine and 5.3% at the hip. The FREEDOM Extension Trial showed that after patients stopped taking Prolia, their fracture risk returned to levels similar to those who had never taken Prolia. Published studies have proven that Prolia is safe to take for at least 8 consecutive years. If your medical provider recommends that you stop taking Prolia, you will need to transition to another osteoporosis medication to maintain the bone protective effects of Prolia.

The bottom line on using Prolia to treat osteoporosis...

Prolia is an antibody created to block the communication signal between osteoblasts and osteoclasts that leads to increased bone breakdown. In doing so, it allows the bone building osteoblasts to catch up in laying new bone – resulting in increased bone density and decreased risk of fracture. Long term studies have shown this medication to be safe and effective for at least 8 years. However, patients with advanced kidney disease and those on dialysis require close monitoring of blood calcium levels in order to prevent hypocalcemia. Patients with weakened immune systems due to medical conditions or use of certain medications including oral steroids require close monitoring for signs and symptoms of infection, which should be treated early to avoid more significant infections requiring hospitalization. Lastly, patients with poor oral hygiene requiring dental extractions are at increased risk of developing osteonecrosis of the jaw. Routine dental screenings and maintaining excellent oral hygiene will minimize the risk of developing osteonecrosis of the jaw. Prolia's convenient twice yearly dosing and significant impact on bone density make it an increasingly more popular option to treat osteoporosis.

13 | Teriparatide (Forteo)

GENERIC NAME	TERIPARATIDE
BRAND NAME	FORTEO
ROUTE	SELF-ADMINISTERED INJECTION INTO THE SUBCUTANEOUS SKIN TISSUE
DOSE	20 MCG DAILY

How does Forteo treat osteoporosis?

Forteo is a medication used to treat osteoporosis, and has also been used off label to aid in fracture healing and as an adjunct treatment for osteonecrosis of the jaw.[139] This medication was designed to mimic the effect that parathyroid hormone has within our body.[140] You may be thinking to yourself... why would you use parathyroid hormone to treat osteoporosis when I previously told you that hyperparathyroidism (elevated levels of parathyroid hormone) can actually CAUSE osteoporosis? Kudos to you for catching this! So how exactly does Forteo work?

The difference lies in the fact that patients with hyperparathyroidism have CONSTANTLY elevated levels of parathyroid hormone. Over time, this can lead to calcium being pulled from our bones! With Forteo, there is a TEMPORARY increase in parathyroid hormone which lasts only a few hours following each daily injection. This temporary increase is associated with increased bone turnover – that is, both increased osteoblast activity and osteoclast activity.[141] Early in the course of treatment, the number of osteoblast cells and the **rate of new bone formation far exceeds osteoclast bone breakdown activity.**[142,143] This leads to new, healthy bone being formed throughout the skeletal system.[141] New bone formation peaks at 6 months after starting Forteo.[142] After 18-24 months, osteoclast function increases to reestablish an equilibrium with osteoblast cells, leading to a plateau in the rate of new bone being formed.[142-144] Long term use of Forteo beyond 2 years is not recommended because the bone-forming effects have run their course and no additional improvement in bone density is achieved.

How effective is Forteo at treating osteoporosis?

When evaluating any treatment for osteoporosis, we must critically evaluate whether the medication improves bone density and decreases the risk of sustaining a fracture. Let's review some of the pertinent studies evaluating the effectiveness of Forteo in the management of osteoporosis.

BONE DENSITY IN WOMEN. A number of studies dating back to the early 2000s have evaluated the effect of Forteo on bone density. In the Fracture Prevention Trial, 1638 postmenopausal women with confirmed osteoporosis and prior spine fractures received either Forteo or a placebo (calcium 1000 mg and vitamin D 400-1200 IU daily).[145] Patients were evaluated over an 18 month period and those receiving 20 mcg of Forteo daily experienced **an increase in bone density of 9% at the spine and 3% at the hip compared to the placebo group**.

BONE DENSITY IN MEN. A separate study was performed to evaluate the effect of Forteo on bone density in men.[146] A total of 437 men between the ages of 30 and 85 with low bone density (T-score -2.0 or lower) were given Forteo or a placebo (1000 mg of calcium and 400-1200 IU vitamin D daily) for approximately 1 year. The patients taking Forteo experienced an **increased bone density of 5.9% at the spine and 1.5% at the hip compared to the placebo group**. This trial was cut short after researchers discovered an increased incidence of a particular type of bone cancer called osteosarcoma in a rat species receiving very high doses of the medication. The risk of osteosarcoma had not been thoroughly evaluated in humans at that time, and the decision to stop the trial simply indicated that more information was needed before further testing could resume in humans.

FRACTURE RISK. Data pulled from the Fracture Prevention Trial also provides insight into the effect of Forteo on the risk of sustaining a fracture. Following the 18 month trial, there was a **65% decreased risk of sustaining a new spine fracture and a 90% decreased risk of sustaining a severe spine fracture compared to the placebo group**. Throughout the duration of the study, it was determined that 14% of patients receiving the placebo experienced a spine fracture, whereas only 5% of patients taking Forteo experienced a spine fracture. Patients taking Forteo were 53% less likely to sustain a non-spine fracture compared to the placebo group.

FORTEO COMPARED TO FOSAMAX IN PATIENTS TAKING ORAL STEROIDS. Treating osteoporosis in patients who are taking oral steroids has proven to be difficult. Studies have been performed aiming to determine which medications are best for these patients. A study of 428 women and men taking oral steroids (at least 5mg daily for 3 or more months) was conducted to compare the effects of Forteo and Fosamax.[147] When comparing the effects on bone density at the lumbar spine after 18 months, **patients taking Forteo experienced an increase of 7.2% compared to 3.4% for Fosamax.** When comparing the incidence of spine fractures, only 0.6% of patients taking Forteo experienced a fracture compared to 6.1% of those taking Fosamax. In this high risk population, Forteo was much more effective in reducing the risk of fractures.

RESULTS AT A GLANCE	
DOES FORTEO IMPROVE BONE DENSITY?	Patients taking Forteo experienced a 5.9% to 9% increase in spine bone density, and a 1.5% to 3% increase in hip bone density following only 12 to 18 months of treatment.
DOES FORTEO DECREASE FRACTURE RISK?	Patients taking Forteo had a 65% decreased risk of spine fracture, a 90% decreased risk of severe spine fractures, and a 53% decreased risk of non-spine fractures following 18 months of treatment.

What are the adverse effects of Forteo?

Your medical provider must balance the benefits of the Forteo with the risks associated with use of this medication. Studies spanning the FDA approved two years of treatment have proven Forteo to be a safe and effective medication, however, below is a list of potential side effects which must be carefully considered.

HEADACHE/DIZZINESS. Headache and dizziness were among the most commonly reported side effects of Forteo. In the Fracture Prevention Trial, 9% of people taking Forteo reported these symptoms compared to 6% of those in the placebo group.[145] Other studies have found no significant difference in the incidence of headache or dizziness between patients taking Forteo and a placebo.[146] If you have a history of chronic headaches or dizziness, these symptoms may worsen once you start taking Forteo.

MUSCLE CRAMPING. Muscle cramping is one of the more commonly reported side effects of Forteo. In the Fracture Prevention Trial, 3% of patients receiving Forteo reported muscle cramps, compared to only 1% of placebo patients.[145]

HYPERCALCEMIA. Transient asymptomatic hypercalcemia, or a temporary increase in blood calcium levels that does not cause any symptoms, occurs more frequently in patients taking Forteo. In the Fracture Prevention Trial, blood calcium levels were measured before receiving the medication and again 4-6 hours later. Elevated calcium levels were found in 11% of Forteo patients compared to only 2% of patients taking placebo.[145] Significant hypercalcemia leading to symptoms and even hospitalization is extremely rare and has not been reported in any major clinical trial. However, a handful of case studies have reported this in select patient populations. Your medical provider may recommend monitoring blood calcium levels periodically to ensure that they remain within the normal range. If they become elevated, it may be recommended that you decrease your daily intake of calcium and vitamin D, or switch to an alternative medication to manage osteoporosis.

HYPERCALCIURIA. Mild increases in the amount of calcium that is released in the urine have been observed in patients taking Forteo, but the incidence of hypercalciuria (excessively high urinary calcium excretion outside of the normal range) did not increase.[145] The mild increase in urinary calcium did not cause kidney stones or other physical symptoms.

HYPERURICEMIA. Uric acid is responsible for those painful flares of gout that many people will experience at some point during their lifetime. Forteo may increase blood uric acid levels, which can increase the risk of gout in select patients.[139] Large studies including the Fracture Prevention Trial did not find any significant difference in gout flares between patients taking Forteo and those taking the placebo, but other studies have indicated an increased incidence of gout.[145] Most cases of gout can be treated with oral anti-inflammatories including Ibuprofen. More severe flares may require oral steroids or even cortisone injections.

OSTEOSARCOMA. Osteosarcoma is a rare form of bone cancer which can lead to pain, disability, and even death. Early Forteo studies were cancelled after osteosarcoma was incidentally discovered in a study involving rats. At that point, more research needed to be conducted to prove the safety of Forteo in human patients before any further human trials could resume.

When we look deeper into the rat study, the rats in the trial that developed osteosarcoma were exposed to highly toxic doses of Forteo for a duration of time similar to the lifespan of the rat – doses that humans would never be exposed to.[148] A separate study exposed monkeys to Forteo doses 10-times greater than that recommended for human use, an no instances of osteosarcoma were reported. A thorough review of all studies dating back nearly 20 years has never shown Forteo to increase the risk of osteosarcoma in the human population. To summarize, does Forteo cause osteosarcoma in humans? No – but expect to hear this risk factor routinely discussed among medical providers and patients alike. The general recommendation is to avoid Forteo in patients that are at increased risk of osteosarcoma, including those who have a history of Paget's disease, and those that have been exposed to radiation.

What dose of Forteo is necessary to treat osteoporosis?

Forteo is administered by an injection into the subcutaneous tissue of the skin performed on a daily basis by the patient. The FDA approved dose of Forteo is 20 mcg daily, and it has been approved for 24 months of consecutive use. After that time, you will need to transition to another osteoporosis medication to "lock in" the improved bone strength established by Forteo.

Once I stop taking Forteo, what happens to my bone density and fracture risk?

Forteo has been shown to dramatically increase bone density and decrease the risk of fracture after only 2 years. As seen with estrogens and Prolia, the effects of Forteo are short lived and will ultimately reverse over a 2 year period unless they are preserved by switching to an alternative osteoporosis medication.[149] In the Parathyroid Hormone and Alendronate for Osteoporosis (PaTH) trial, 238 postmenopausal women between the ages of 55 and 85 with documented osteoporosis were treated with 12 months of Forteo followed by either Fosamax or a placebo (calcium and vitamin D supplementation).[150] Over the 2 year trial, **patients who received 12 months of Forteo followed by 12 months of Fosamax had a bone density increase of 12.1% at the spine. Patients who received 12 months of Forteo followed by 12 months of a placebo had only a 4.1% increase in spine bone density**. The findings of this study indicate that switching from Forteo to a bisphosphonate like Fosamax will preserve the bone protective effects of Forteo. Patients who do not transition to another osteoporosis medication following Forteo will lose the bone protective effects of Forteo over a 2 year period.

The bottom line on using Forteo to treat osteoporosis…

Forteo is a synthetic form of parathyroid hormone which is highly effective at increasing bone density and decreasing fracture risk. It works differently than the other osteoporosis medications currently on the market by directly increasing the activity of osteoblasts to lay new healthy bone tissue. Several studies in humans spanning the FDA-approved 24 month duration have proven Forteo to be safe and effective. Patients receiving Forteo were more likely to experience headaches, nausea, and muscle cramping compared to patients receiving the placebo. Blood and urine calcium levels have been shown to increase while taking Forteo, however, unless the patient has an underlying medical condition that predisposes them to such events, it is unlikely that these elevated calcium levels will lead to any symptoms. While the risk of osteosarcoma is frequently a cause of concern for patients, and rightfully so, the medication has never been shown to cause this form of cancer in humans taking prescribed doses. The only study indicating an increased risk of osteosarcoma was in a study with rats receiving highly toxic doses throughout the entire lifespan of the rat – a scenario that provides no useful information for humans. With that said, it is probably still best to avoid this medication in patients at increased risk of developing osteosarcoma, including patients with a history of Paget's disease and those who have previously received radiation treatments for cancer.

Forteo has been shown to have the greatest positive effect on bone density and fracture risk compared to all other treatments on the market… but is it right for you? This is a tough question, and is best answered by your medical provider. Forteo is often reserved for patients with severe osteoporosis, which is defined as a T-score less than -3.5, or patients who have experienced multiple prior osteoporosis-related fractures. Other patients who are excellent candidates include those who have failed other osteoporosis treatments – meaning their bone density continues to decline on follow-up DXA scans, or those who sustain a fracture while on other treatments. While Forteo is not the first treatment for all patients, if your medical provider recommends Forteo, you should strongly consider how this medication can improve your bone health.

14 You've Picked your Treatment... Now What?

You've decided on the best treatment plan for you... now what?

Congratulations! You have taken all of the necessary steps to be proactive about your bone health. You've successfully waded through the mountain of information regarding all of the treatment options and are now armed with all of the facts necessary to choose the plan that best fits your needs. That alone is a cause for celebration! But what happens next? How do you know if the treatment(s) you have chosen is actually improving your bone health? When should you jump ship and consider alternative treatment options? These are excellent questions, and there is no simple answer. When I assess a patient's response to osteoporosis treatments, I consider three variables – changes in DXA scan results, bone turnover markers, and new fractures. I will discuss how each of these variables relates to monitoring your response to treatment below.

BONE DENSITY (DXA). Regardless of which treatment is chosen, it is important to monitor your bone density over time. Most people taking osteoporosis medications will experience a decrease in their fracture risk within a few months; however, it can take 1-2 years before measurable bone density increases show up on DXA scans. Most insurance plans are willing to pay for DXA scans every 2 years, making this a reasonable time to reassess bone density. Ideally, the DXA scan will include two anatomic locations (hip, spine, and/or wrist) and will be performed on the same DXA machine as your prior scan for the most accurate result. **My definition of a treatment success is a bone density that remains the same or improves over a two year period.** If bone density decreases significantly, this could indicate a treatment failure.

BONE TURNOVER MARKERS. If you recall from our previous discussion, bone turnover markers are used to measure the speed at which old bone is recycled and new bone is created. Medications including the bisphosphonates and Prolia decrease the rate of old bone being recycled, allowing for new bone to be formed. Forteo is unique in that it directly increases the rate in which new bone is formed. Certain blood and urine lab tests (CTX, NTX, and P1NP) can measure these changes, and within 3-6 months provide a fairly accurate assessment of whether a medication is working appropriately. **If the bone turnover marker labs change as anticipated following the start of a new treatment, this provides reassurance that the treatment is successful.** If the bone turnover markers DO NOT change as anticipated, this raises the concern that the patient is not responding to treatment.

FRACTURE. The ultimate goal of any osteoporosis treatment is to reduce the incidence of fractures. The medications available have been shown to decrease the rate of sustaining a fracture by as much as 50-75%! While this is impressive, it means that even under the best of circumstances, some patients receiving treatment for osteoporosis will continue to fracture. The initial impulse is to consider fractures a treatment failure. But what if this same patient would have sustained multiple fractures without treatment, and instead only had a single fracture with treatment? Most would consider that a treatment success! We do not have a crystal ball to provide us with these answers, so we must carefully consider other indicators of treatment success before considering new fractures a treatment failure.

After reviewing the three most important variables for determining treatment success, you can appreciate that the decision is not an easy one. My rule of thumb is that failure of any of the above in isolation does not indicate unsuccessful treatment, but if a patient fails two or more variables, then other treatment options must be considered.

Let's consider a few examples to illustrate my point. Our first patient is Dorothy, a 65 year old female without a prior fracture but with osteoporosis. She made the decision to start taking Fosamax 2 years ago – her bone turnover markers decreased within 6 months and her follow up DXA scan showed that her bone density improved! However, she recently fell and sustained a wrist fracture. In this scenario, she has shown excellent response to treatment in two of the variables – bone turnover markers decreased and bone density increased. She did sustain a recent fracture, but this would not be considered a treatment failure because her other variables all point to a treatment success!

Our next patient is Mary. She is 59 years old and has a history of a prior spine compression fracture and a significant family history of osteoporosis. She was started on Prolia and her bone turnover markers after 6 months of treatment decreased, indicating successful treatment! However, her DXA scan showed that her bone density had slightly worsened. She continued with Prolia, but experienced sudden low back pain and another spine compression fracture! She has now failed two variables – her bone density did not improve on the medication AND she sustained a fracture. This would be considered a treatment failure and I would recommend considering alternative treatment options to better protect her bones.

Our final patient is Jake. He is a 70 year old male who was diagnosed with osteoporosis after he sustained a hip fracture. He was started on Reclast, but never had his bone turnover markers measured. His bone density improved on his follow up DXA scan, however, he sustained a spine compression fracture 2 years after starting treatment. This scenario is more difficult to assess because we only have two variables to assess. His bone density improved, but he continued to fracture… so is this a failure or not? With an improvement in bone density, I would lean toward a treatment success and closely monitor him in the future. If he had ANOTHER fracture, then switching to an alternative treatment would be strongly considered. Ultimately, only the patient and the medical provider can determine which treatment is most appropriate.

My Parting Words

By simply reading this book you have already taken the first and most important step towards improving your bone health. You are now armed with all of the necessary information to have an educated discussion regarding osteoporosis with your medical provider. Together, you can select the treatment that is most appropriate for your personal needs. And don't be selfish with your newfound knowledge! Share this information with your family, friends, coworkers, strangers, pets, inanimate objects, and anyone who will listen! How empowering is it to know that YOU could prevent the unnecessary pain and suffering of fractures from osteoporosis? Osteoporosis is a widespread disease that affects millions of people throughout the world – with your help, we can make a difference!

15 Patient Osteoporosis Questionnaire

1) Have you experienced menopause? If so, at what age?
2) Personal history of low trauma fracture?
3) Personal history of stress fracture?
4) Family history of osteoporosis or low trauma fracture?
5) Number of falls in last year?
6) History of smoking or use of tobacco products?
7) Do you consume more than 2 alcoholic beverages daily?
8) Have you ever been diagnosed with high or low calcium/vitamin D?
9) Do you currently supplement calcium or vitamin D? If so, at what doses?
10) Do you currently weigh <127 pounds?
11) Have you ever been diagnosed with any of the following medical conditions?
    - Hyperthyroidism
    - Hyperparathyroidism
    - Celiac disease
    - Hypercalciuria (elevated calcium in the urine)
    - Multiple myeloma
    - Cushing's disease
    - Hypogonadism
    - Kidney or liver disease
    - Rheumatoid arthritis
    - Diabetes: Type I or II
12) Have you taken any of the following medications?
    - Aromatase Inhibitors: Anastrazole, Letrozole, Exemestrane
    - Antidepressants: Zoloft, Celexa, Prozac
    - Anti-epileptic Drugs: Carbamazepine, Valproate, Phenobarbital, Phenytoin
    - Calcineurin Inhibitors: Cyclosporine, Tacrolimus
    - Depot medroxyprogesterone acetate
    - Glucocorticoids: Prednisone
    - GnRH Agonists: Leuprorelin, Triptorelin, Goserelin,
    - Proton Pump Inhibitors: Protonix, Nexium, Prevacid
    - Thiazolidinediones: Avandia

16   Treatment of Osteoporosis

1) Smoking Cessation

2) Avoid excessive alcohol consumption of greater than 2 drinks per day

3) Weight bearing Exercise
- Weight bearing exercises have been shown to improve bone strength, improve muscle strength, and decrease the risk of falls
- You should participate in weight bearing exercises for a minimum of 30 minutes three times weekly
- Exercises include walking, hiking, dancing, yoga, golf, racquet sports, and strength training

4) Calcium
- Calcium is an essential mineral that is needed to build strong bones
- Dosing Requirements
  - Pre-menopausal women: **800-1000** mg daily
  - Post-menopausal women and all men: **1200** mg daily
  - Maximum intake: avoid consuming more than 2000 mg daily
  - Half of daily calcium intake should come from dietary sources
- Calcium supplements come in two forms: calcium carbonate and calcium citrate
  - Calcium carbonate should be taken with food, while calcium citrate can be taken with food or fasting
  - Calcium citrate is preferred if you take proton pump inhibitors or other acid reducers
- Dietary sources of calcium
  - 300 mg per serving: 8 oz. milk/yogurt, 1 oz. hard cheese
  - 150 mg per serving: 4 oz. cottage cheese/ice cream
  - 100-200 mg per serving: dark green vegetables, nuts, breads, fortified cereals

5) Vitamin D
- Vitamin D enhances your body's ability to absorb calcium and build strong bones
- Dosing Requirements
  - Pre-menopausal women: **600** IU daily

- o Post-menopausal women and all men: **800-1000** IU daily
- o Maximum intake: avoid consuming more than 4000 IU daily unless directed by your physician
- Vitamin D comes in two forms: Vitamin D3 (cholecalciferol) and Vitamin D2 (ergocalciferol)
  - o Both forms of Vitamin D can be taken fasting or with meals
  - o Both Vitamin D3 and Vitamin D2 are well absorbed by the body and neither is preferred
- Sources of Vitamin D
  - o Commercially fortified milk: 100 IU/8oz.
  - o Cod liver oil
  - o Mushrooms exposed to sunlight
  - o Sunlight exposure (UVB)

6) Osteoporosis Medications
- Medications approved by the FDA for the treatment of osteoporosis include Estrogens, Bisphosphonates, Prolia, and Forteo.

References

1. Cooper, C., Campion, G., & Melton III, L. (1992). Hip fractures in the elderly: a world-wide projection. *Osteoporosis international, 2*(6), 285-289.

2. General, S. (2004). Bone health and osteoporosis: a report of the surgeon general. *US Department of Health and Human Services, Office of the Surgeon General, Rockville, MD.*

3. Melton, L. J., Chrischilles, E. A., Cooper, C., Lane, A. W., & Riggs, B. L. (2005). How many women have osteoporosis?. *Journal of bone and mineral research, 20*(5), 886-892.

4. Randell, A., Nguyen, T. V., Lapsley, H., Jones, G., Kelly, P. J., & Eisman, J. A. (1995). Direct clinical and welfare costs of osteoporotic fractures in elderly men and women. *Osteoporosis International, 5*(6), 427-432.

5. Johnell, O., & Kanis, J. A. (2006). An estimate of the worldwide prevalence and disability associated with osteoporotic fractures. *Osteoporosis international, 17*(12), 1726-1733.

6. Kanis, J. A., Johnell, O., De Laet, C., Johansson, H., Odén, A., Delmas, P., & McCloskey, E. V. (2004). A meta-analysis of previous fracture and subsequent fracture risk. *Bone, 35*(2), 375-382.

7. Gullberg, B., Johnell, O., & Kanis, J. A. (1997). World-wide projections for hip fracture. *Osteoporosis international, 7*(5), 407-413.

8. Kostenuik, P. J. (2005). Osteoprotegerin and RANKL regulate bone resorption, density, geometry and strength. *Current opinion in pharmacology, 5*(6), 618-625.

9. Baxter-Jones, A. D., Faulkner, R. A., Forwood, M. R., Mirwald, R. L., & Bailey, D. A. (2011). Bone mineral accrual from 8 to 30 years of age: an estimation of peak bone mass. *Journal of bone and mineral research, 26*(8), 1729-1739.

10. Stepan, J. J., Alenfeld, F., Boivin, G., Feyen, J. H., & Lakatos, P. (2003). Mechanisms of action of antiresorptive therapies of postmenopausal osteoporosis. *Endocrine regulations, 37*(4), 225-238.

11. Recker, R., Lappe, J., Davies, K., & Heaney, R. (2000). Characterization of perimenopausal bone loss: a prospective study. *Journal of Bone and Mineral Research, 15*(10), 1965-1973.

12. Hannan, M. T., Felson, D. T., Dawson-Hughes, B., Tucker, K. L., Cupples, L. A., Wilson, P. W., & Kiel, D. P. (2000). Risk factors for longitudinal bone loss in elderly men and women: the Framingham Osteoporosis Study. *Journal of Bone and Mineral Research, 15*(4), 710-720.

13. Kanis, J. A., Johansson, H., Johnell, O., Oden, A., De Laet, C., Eisman, J. A., & Tenenhouse, A. (2005). Alcohol intake as a risk factor for fracture. *Osteoporosis international, 16*(7), 737-742.

14. Hopper, J. L., & Seeman, E. (1994). The bone density of female twins discordant for tobacco use. *New England Journal of Medicine, 330*(6), 387-392.

15. Kanis, J. A., Johnell, O., Odén, A., Johansson, H., De Laet, C., Eisman, J. A., & Melton, L. J. (2005). Smoking and fracture risk: a meta-analysis. *Osteoporosis International, 16*(2), 155-162.

16. Riggs, B. L., & Melton III, L. J. (1986). Involutional osteoporosis. *New England journal of medicine, 314*(26), 1676-1686.

17. Gallagher JC: Osteoporosis. Conn's Current Therapy. Robert ER (ed). Philadelphia, WB Saunders Co, 1999, pp 590-594

18. Ryan, C. S., Petkov, V. I., & Adler, R. A. (2011). Osteoporosis in men: the value of laboratory testing. *Osteoporosis International, 22*(6), 1845-1853.

19. Painter, S. E., Kleerekoper, M., & Camacho, P. M. (2006). Secondary osteoporosis: a review of the recent evidence. *Endocrine Practice, 12*(4), 436-445.

20. Tannenbaum, C., Clark, J., Schwartzman, K., Wallenstein, S., Lapinski, R., Meier, D., & Luckey, M. (2002). Yield of laboratory testing to identify secondary contributors to osteoporosis in otherwise healthy women. *The Journal of Clinical Endocrinology & Metabolism, 87*(10), 4431-4437.

21. Ryan, C. S., Petkov, V. I., & Adler, R. A. (2011). Osteoporosis in men: the value of laboratory testing. *Osteoporosis International, 22*(6), 1845-1853.

22. Painter, S. E., Kleerekoper, M., & Camacho, P. M. (2006). Secondary osteoporosis: a review of the recent evidence. *Endocrine Practice, 12*(4), 436-445.

23. Tannenbaum, C., Clark, J., Schwartzman, K., Wallenstein, S., Lapinski, R., Meier, D., & Luckey, M. (2002). Yield of laboratory testing to identify secondary contributors to osteoporosis in otherwise healthy women. *The Journal of Clinical Endocrinology & Metabolism, 87*(10), 4431-4437.

24. Nicodemus, K. K., & Folsom, A. R. (2001). Type 1 and type 2 diabetes and incident hip fractures in postmenopausal women. *Diabetes care, 24*(7), 1192-1197.

25. Bassett, J. D., O'Shea, P. J., Sriskantharajah, S., Rabier, B., Boyde, A., Howell, P. G., & Samarut, J. (2007). Thyroid hormone excess rather than thyrotropin deficiency induces osteoporosis in hyperthyroidism. *Molecular Endocrinology, 21*(5), 1095-1107.

26. Bauer, D. C., Ettinger, B., Nevitt, M. C., & Stone, K. L. (2001). Risk for fracture in women with low serum levels of thyroid-stimulating hormone. *Annals of Internal Medicine, 134*(7), 561-568.

27. Grey, A., Mitnick, M. A., Shapses, S., Ellison, A. Gundberg, C., & Insogna, K. (1996). Circulating levels of interleukin-6 and tumor necrosis factor-alpha are elevated in primary hyperparathyroidism and correlate with markers of bone resorption--a clinical research center study. *The Journal of Clinical Endocrinology & Metabolism, 81*(10), 3450-3454.

28. Pasieka, J. L., Parsons, L. L., Demeure, M. J., Wilson, S., Malycha, P., Jones, J., & Krzywda, B. (2002). Patient-based surgical outcome tool demonstrating alleviation of symptoms following parathyroidectomy in patients with primary hyperparathyroidism. *World journal of surgery, 26*(8), 942-949.

29. Giannini, S., Nobile, M., Sella, S., Carbonare, L. D., & Favus, M. J. (2005). Bone disease in primary hypercalciuria. *Critical reviews in clinical laboratory sciences, 42*(3), 229-248.

30. Adams, J. S., Song, C. F., & Kantorovich, V. (1999). Rapid recovery of bone mass in hypercalciuric, osteoporotic men treated with hydrochlorothiazide. *Annals of internal medicine, 130*(8), 658-660.

31. Khosla S, Amin S, Orwoll E (2008) Osteoporosis in men. *Endocr Rev* **29**: 441-64.

32. Stenson, W. F., Newberry, R., Lorenz, R., Baldus, C., & Civitelli, R. (2005). Increased prevalence of celiac disease and need for routine screening among patients with osteoporosis. *Archives of Internal Medicine, 165*(4), 393-399.

33. Sezer, O., Heider, U., Zavrski, I., Kühne, C. A., & Hofbauer, L. C. (2003). RANK ligand and osteoprotegerin in myeloma bone disease. *Blood, 101*(6), 2094-2098.

34. Tian, E., Zhan, F., Walker, R., Rasmussen, E., Ma, Y., Barlogie, B., & Shaughnessy Jr, J. D. (2003). The role of the Wnt-signaling antagonist DKK1 in the development of osteolytic lesions in multiple myeloma. *New England Journal of Medicine, 349*(26), 2483-2494.

35. Barete, S., Assous, N., De Gennes, C., Grandpeix, C., Feger, F., Palmerini, F., & Fraitag, S. (2010). Systemic mastocytosis and bone involvement in a cohort of 75 patients. *Annals of the rheumatic diseases, 69*(10), 1838-1841.

36. Chiappetta, N., & Gruber, B. (2006, August). The role of mast cells in osteoporosis. In *Seminars in arthritis and rheumatism* (Vol. 36, No. 1, pp. 32-36). WB Saunders.

37. Geisler, J., & Lønning, P. E. (2010). Impact of aromatase inhibitors on bone health in breast cancer patients. *The Journal of steroid biochemistry and molecular biology, 118*(4), 294-299.

38. Hadji, Peyman. "Aromatase inhibitor-associated bone loss in breast cancer patients is distinct from postmenopausal osteoporosis." *Critical reviews in oncology/hematology* 69.1 (2009): 73-82.

39. Rizzoli, R., Cooper, C., Reginster, J. Y., Abrahamsen, B., Adachi, J. D., Brandi, M. L., & Harvey, N. C. (2012). Antidepressant medications and osteoporosis. *Bone, 51*(3), 606-613.

40. Rivelli, S. K., & Muzyk, A. J. (2009). Antidepressants and Osteoporosis. *Psychopharm Review, 44*(8), 57-63.

41. Chung, S., & Ahn, C. (1994). Effects of anti-epileptic drug therapy on bone mineral density in ambulatory epileptic children. *Brain and Development, 16*(5), 382-385.

42. Sheth, R. D., Wesolowski, C. A., Jacob, J. C., Penney, S., Hobbs, G. R., Riggs, J. E., & Bodensteiner, J. B. (1995). Effect of carbamazepine and valproate on bone mineral density. *The Journal of pediatrics, 127*(2), 256-262.

43. Nakken, K. O., & Taubøll, E. (2010). Bone loss associated with use of antiepileptic drugs. *Expert opinion on drug safety, 9*(4), 561-571.

44. Movsowitz, C., Epstein, S., Fallon, M. E. A., Ismail, F., & Thomas, S. (1988). Cyclosporin-A in Vivo Produces Severe Osteopenia in the Rat: Effect of Dose and Duration of Administration*. *Endocrinology, 123*(5), 2571-2577.

45. Edwards, B. J., Desai, A., Tsai, J., Du, H., Edwards, G. R., Bunta, A. D., & Sprague, S. (2011). Elevated incidence of fractures in solid-organ transplant recipients on glucocorticoid-sparing immunosuppressive regimens. *Journal of osteoporosis, 2011*.

46. Kaunitz, A. M., Arias, R., & McClung, M. (2008). Bone density recovery after depot medroxyprogesterone acetate injectable contraception use. *Contraception, 77*(2), 67-76.

47. Meier, C., Brauchli, Y. B., Jick, S. S., Kraenzlin, M. E., & Meier, C. R. (2010). Use of depot medroxyprogesterone acetate and fracture risk. *The Journal of Clinical Endocrinology & Metabolism, 95*(11), 4909-4916.

48. Thorstenson, A., Bratt, O., Akre, O., Hellborg, H., Holmberg, L., Lambe, M., & Adolfsson, J. (2012). Incidence of fractures causing hospitalisation in prostate cancer patients: results from the population-based PCBaSe Sweden. *European Journal of Cancer, 48*(11), 1672-1681.

49. Ngamruengphong, S., Leontiadis, G. I., Radhi, S., Dentino, A., & Nugent, K. (2011). Proton pump inhibitors and risk of fracture: a systematic review and meta-analysis of observational studies. *The American journal of gastroenterology, 106*(7), 1209-1218.

50. Lecka-Czernik, B. (2010). Bone loss in diabetes: use of antidiabetic thiazolidinediones and secondary osteoporosis. *Current osteoporosis reports, 8*(4), 178-184.

51. Meier, C., Kraenzlin, M. E., Bodmer, M., Jick, S. S., Jick, H., & Meier, C. R. (2008). Use of thiazolidinediones and fracture risk. *Archives of Internal Medicine, 168*(8), 820-825.

52. Fraser, L. A., & Adachi, J. D. (2009). Glucocorticoid-induced osteoporosis: treatment update and review. *Therapeutic advances in musculoskeletal disease, 1*(2), 71-85.

53. Canalis, E., Mazziotti, G., Giustina, A., & Bilezikian, J. P. (2007). Glucocorticoid-induced osteoporosis: pathophysiology and therapy. *Osteoporosis International, 18*(10), 1319-1328.

54. Schousboe, J. T., Shepherd, J. A., Bilezikian, J. P., & Baim, S. (2013). Executive summary of the 2013 international society for clinical densitometry position development conference on bone densitometry. *Journal of Clinical Densitometry, 16*(4), 455-466.

55. Gourlay, M. L., Fine, J. P., Preisser, J. S., May, R. C., Li, C., Lui, L. Y., & Ensrud, K. E. (2012). Bone-density testing interval and transition to osteoporosis in older women. *New England Journal of Medicine, 366*(3), 225-233.

56. Worsfold, M., Powell, D. E., Jones, T. J., & Davie, M. W. (2004). Assessment of urinary bone markers for monitoring treatment of osteoporosis. *Clinical chemistry, 50*(12), 2263-2270.

57. Delmas, P. D., Eastell, R., Garnero, P., Seibel, M. J., & Stepan, J. (2000). The use of biochemical markers of bone turnover in osteoporosis. *Osteoporosis International, 11*(18), S2-S17.

58. Eastell, R., Krege, J. H., Chen, P., Glass, E. V., & Reginster, J. Y. (2005). Development of an algorithm for using PINP to monitor treatment of patients with teriparatide*. *Current Medical Research and Opinion®, 22*(1), 61-66.

59. Kanis, J. A., McCloskey, E. V., Johansson, H., Strom, O., Borgstrom, F., & Odén, A. (2008). Case finding for the management of osteoporosis with FRAX®—assessment and intervention thresholds for the UK. *Osteoporosis international, 19*(10), 1395-1408.

60. Looker, A. C., Orwoll, E. S., Johnston, C. C., Lindsay, R. L., Wahner, H. W., Dunn, W. L., & Heyse, S. P. (1997). Prevalence of low femoral bone density in

older US adults from NHANES III. *Journal of Bone and Mineral Research*, *12*(11), 1761-1768.

61. Ryan, C. S., Petkov, V. I., & Adler, R. A. (2011). Osteoporosis in men: the value of laboratory testing. *Osteoporosis International*, *22*(6), 1845-1853.

62. Burge, R., Dawson-Hughes, B., Solomon, D. H., Wong, J. B., King, A., & Tosteson, A. (2007). Incidence and economic burden of osteoporosis-related fractures in the United States, 2005–2025. *Journal of bone and mineral research*, *22*(3), 465-475.

63. Kiebzak, G. M., Beinart, G. A., Perser, K., Ambrose, C. G., Siff, S. J., & Heggeness, M. H. (2002). Undertreatment of osteoporosis in men with hip fracture. *Archives of Internal Medicine*, *162*(19), 2217-2222.

64. Kanis, J. A., Melton, L. 3., Christiansen, C., Johnston, C. C., & Khaltaev, N. (1994). The diagnosis of osteoporosis. *J Bone Miner Res*, *9*(8), 1137-1141.

65. Lewiecki, E. M., Watts, N. B., McClung, M. R., Petak, S. M., Bachrach, L. K., Shepherd, J. A., & Downs Jr, R. W. (2004). Official positions of the international society for clinical densitometry. *The Journal of Clinical Endocrinology & Metabolism*, *89*(8), 3651-3655.

66. Looker, A. C., Orwoll, E. S., Johnston, C. C., Lindsay, R. L., Wahner, H. W., Dunn, W. L., & Heyse, S. P. (1997). Prevalence of low femoral bone density in older US adults from NHANES III. *Journal of Bone and Mineral Research*, *12*(11), 1761-1768.

67. Melton, L. J., Chrischilles, E. A., Cooper, C., Lane, A. W., & Riggs, B. L. (2005). How many women have osteoporosis?. *Journal of bone and mineral research*, *20*(5), 886-892.

68. Cosman, F., De Beur, S. J., LeBoff, M. S., Lewiecki, E. M., Tanner, B., Randall, S., & Lindsay, R. (2014). Clinician's guide to prevention and treatment of osteoporosis. *Osteoporosis international*, *25*(10), 2359-2381.

69. The Writing Group for the ISCD Position Development Conference. (2004). Diagnosis of osteoporosis in men, premenopausal women, and children. *Journal of Clinical Densitometry*, *7*(1), 17-26.

70. Díez-Pérez, A., Hooven, F. H., Adachi, J. D., Adami, S., Anderson, F. A., Boonen, S., & Greenspan, S. L. (2011). Regional differences in treatment for osteoporosis. The Global Longitudinal Study of Osteoporosis in Women (GLOW). *Bone*, *49*(3), 493-498.

71. Fraser, L. A., & Adachi, J. D. (2009). Glucocorticoid-induced osteoporosis: treatment update and review. *Therapeutic advances in musculoskeletal disease*, *1*(2), 71-85.

72. Canalis, E., Mazziotti, G., Giustina, A., & Bilezikian, J. P. (2007). Glucocorticoid-induced osteoporosis: pathophysiology and therapy. *Osteoporosis International*, *18*(10), 1319-1328.

73. Van Staa, T. P., Leufkens, H. G. M., Abenhaim, L., Zhang, B., & Cooper, C. (2000). Use of oral corticosteroids and risk of fractures. *Journal of Bone and Mineral Research*, *15*(6), 993-1000.

74. Homik, J., Cranney, A., Shea, B., Tugwell, P., Wells, G., & Adachi, R. (2000). Bisphosphonates for steroid induced osteoporosis (Cochrane Review) The Cochrane Library, Issue 3, Update Software.

75. Saag, K. G., Shane, E., Boonen, S., Marín, F., Donley, D. W., Taylor, K. A., & Marcus, R. (2007). Teriparatide or Alendronate in glucocorticoid-induced osteoporosis. *New England Journal of Medicine, 357*(20), 2028-2039.

76. MacLean, C., Newberry, S., Maglione, M., McMahon, M., Ranganath, V., Suttorp, M., & Desai, S. B. (2008). Systematic review: comparative effectiveness of treatments to prevent fractures in men and women with low bone density or osteoporosis. *Annals of Internal Medicine, 148*(3), 197-213.

77. Wysocki, A., Butler, M., Shamliyan, T., & Kane, R. L. (2011). Whole-body vibration therapy for osteoporosis: state of the science. *Annals of internal medicine, 155*(10), 680-686.

78. Howe, T. E., Shea, B., Dawson, L. J., Downie, F., Murray, A., Ross, C., & Creed, G. (2011). Exercise for preventing and treating osteoporosis in postmenopausal women. *The Cochrane Library*.

79. Nordin, B. C. (1997). Calcium and osteoporosis. *Nutrition, 13*(7), 664-686.

80. Potts, J. T., & Gardella, T. J. (2011). Parathyroid Hormone and Calcium Homeostasis. *Pediatric Bone: Biology & Diseases*, 109.

81. NIH Concensus Panel (1994). NIH Consensus Conference. Optimal calcium intake. NIH consensus development panel on optimal calcium intake. *JAMA, 272*, 1942-1948.

82. Straub, D. A. (2007). Calcium supplementation in clinical practice: a review of forms, doses, and indications. *Nutrition in Clinical Practice, 22*(3), 286-296.

83. Curhan, G. C., Willett, W. C., Speizer, F. E., Spiegelman, D., & Stampfer, M. J. (1997). Comparison of dietary calcium with supplemental calcium and other nutrients as factors affecting the risk for kidney stones in women. *Annals of Internal Medicine, 126*(7), 497-504.

84. Bolland, M. J., Avenell, A., Baron, J. A., Grey, A., MacLennan, G. S., Gamble, G. D., & Reid, I. R. (2010). Effect of calcium supplements on risk of myocardial infarction and cardiovascular events: meta-analysis. *Bmj, 341*, c3691.

85. Li, K., Kaaks, R., Linseisen, J., & Rohrmann, S. (2012). Associations of dietary calcium intake and calcium supplementation with myocardial infarction and stroke risk and overall cardiovascular mortality in the Heidelberg cohort of the European Prospective Investigation into Cancer and Nutrition study (EPIC-Heidelberg). *Heart, 98*(12), 920-925.

86. Murad, M. H., Elamin, K. B., Abu Elnour, N. O., Elamin, M. B., Alkatib, A. A., Fatourechi, M. M., & Erwin, P. J. (2011). The effect of vitamin D on falls: a systematic review and meta-analysis. *The Journal of Clinical Endocrinology & Metabolism, 96*(10), 2997-3006.

87. Pfeifer, Michael, et al. "Effects of a short-term vitamin D and calcium supplementation on body sway and secondary hyperparathyroidism in elderly women." *Journal of Bone and Mineral Research* 15.6 (2000): 1113-1118.

88. Holick, M. F., Binkley, N. C., Bischoff-Ferrari, H. A., Gordon, C. M., Hanley, D. A., Heaney, R. P., ... & Weaver, C. M. (2011). Evaluation, treatment, and prevention of vitamin D deficiency: an Endocrine Society clinical practice guideline. *The Journal of Clinical Endocrinology & Metabolism, 96*(7), 1911-1930.

89. Forrest, K. Y., & Stuhldreher, W. L. (2011). Prevalence and correlates of vitamin D deficiency in US adults. *Nutrition research*, *31*(1), 48-54.

90. Holick, M. F., Biancuzzo, R. M., Chen, T. C., Klein, E. K., Young, A., Bibuld, D., & Tannenbaum, A. D. (2008). Vitamin D2 is as effective as vitamin D3 in maintaining circulating concentrations of 25-hydroxyvitamin D. *The Journal of Clinical Endocrinology & Metabolism*, *93*(3), 677-681.

91. Tuohimaa, P., Lyakhovich, A., Aksenov, N., Pennanen, P., Syvälä, H., Lou, Y. R., & Manninen, T. (2001). Vitamin D and prostate cancer. *The Journal of steroid biochemistry and molecular biology*, *76*(1), 125-134.

92. Holick, M. F., Binkley, N. C., Bischoff-Ferrari, H. A., Gordon, C. M., Hanley, D. A., Heaney, R. P., ... & Weaver, C. M. (2012). Guidelines for preventing and treating vitamin D deficiency and insufficiency revisited. *The Journal of Clinical Endocrinology & Metabolism*, *97*(4), 1153-1158.

93. Jackson, R. D., LaCroix, A. Z., Gass, M., Wallace, R. B., Robbins, J., Lewis, C. E., & Bonds, D. E. (2006). Calcium plus vitamin D supplementation and the risk of fractures. *New England Journal of Medicine*, *354*(7), 669-683.

94. Stepan, J. J., Alenfeld, F., Boivin, G., Feyen, J. H., & Lakatos, P. (2003). Mechanisms of action of antiresorptive therapies of postmenopausal osteoporosis. *Endocrine regulations*, *37*(4), 225-238.

95. Jacobsen, D. E., Samson, M. M., Kezic, S., & Verhaar, H. J. J. (2007). Postmenopausal HRT and tibolone in relation to muscle strength and body composition. *Maturitas*, *58*(1), 7-18.

96. Naessen, T., Lindmark, B., & Larsen, H. C. (2007). Hormone therapy and postural balance in elderly women. *Menopause*, *14*(6), 1020-1024.

97. Bea, J. W., Zhao, Q., Cauley, J. A., LaCroix, A. Z., Bassford, T., Lewis, C. E., & Chen, Z. (2011). Effect of hormone therapy on lean body mass, falls, and fractures: Six-year results from the Women's Health Initiative Hormone Trials. *Menopause (New York, NY)*, *18*(1), 44.

98. Bolscher, M., Netelenbos, J. C., Barto, R., & van Buuren, L. M. (1999). Estrogen regulation of intestinal calcium absorption in the intact and ovariectomized adult rat. *Journal of Bone and Mineral Research*, *14*(7), 1197-1202.

99. Wells, G., Tugwell, P., Shea, B., Guyatt, G., Peterson, J., Zytaruk, N., & Cranney, A. (2002). V. Meta-analysis of the efficacy of hormone replacement therapy in treating and preventing osteoporosis in postmenopausal women. *Endocrine Reviews*, *23*(4), 529-539.

100. Rossouw JE *et al.* (2004) Risks and benefits of estrogen plus progestin in healthy postmenopausal women: principle results from the Women's Health Initiative randomized controlled trial. *JAMA* **288**(3): 321-33.

101. La Vecchia, C., Brinton, L. A., & McTiernan, A. (2002). Cancer risk in menopausal women. *Best Practice & Research Clinical Obstetrics & Gynaecology*, *16*(3), 293-307.

102. Ziel, H. K., & Finkle, W. D. (1975). Increased risk of endometrial carcinoma among users of conjugated estrogens. *New England journal of medicine*, *293*(23), 1167-1170.

103. Grady, D., Gebretsadik, T., Kerlikowske, K., Ernster, V., & Petitti, D. (1995). Hormone replacement therapy and endometrial cancer risk: a meta-analysis. *Obstetrics & Gynecology*, *85*(2), 304-313.

104. Canonico, M., Plu-Bureau, G., Lowe, G. D., & Scarabin, P. Y. (2008). Hormone replacement therapy and risk of venous thromboembolism in postmenopausal women: systematic review and meta-analysis. *Bmj*, *336*(7655), 1227-1231.

105. Cirillo, D. J., Wallace, R. B., Rodabough, R. J., Greenland, P., LaCroix, A. Z., Limacher, M. C., & Larson, J. C. (2005). Effect of estrogen therapy on gallbladder disease. *Jama*, *293*(3), 330-339.

106. Grodstein F, Manson JE, Stampfer MJ, Rexrode K 2008 Postmenopausal hormone therapy and stroke: role of time since menopause and age at initiation of hormone therapy. Arch Intern Med 168:861–866

107. Banks, E., Beral, V., Reeves, G., Balkwill, A., Barnes, I., & Million Women Study Collaborators. (2004). Fracture incidence in relation to the pattern of use of hormone therapy in postmenopausal women. *Jama*, *291*(18), 2212-2220.

108. Nancollas, G. H., Tang, R., Phipps, R. J., Henneman, Z., Gulde, S., Wu, W., & Ebetino, F. H. (2006). Novel insights into actions of bisphosphonates on bone: differences in interactions with hydroxyapatite. *Bone*, *38*(5), 617-627.

109. Rodan, G. A., Seedor, J. G., & Balena, R. (1993). Preclinical pharmacology of Alendronate. *Osteoporosis international*, *3*(3), 7-12.

110. Russell, R. G. G., Watts, N. B., Ebetino, F. H., & Rogers, M. J. (2008). Mechanisms of action of bisphosphonates: similarities and differences and their potential influence on clinical efficacy. *Osteoporosis international*, *19*(6), 733-759.

111. Ebetino, F. H., Hogan, A. M. L., Sun, S., Tsoumpra, M. K., Duan, X., Triffitt, J. T., & Lundy, M. W. (2011). The relationship between the chemistry and biological activity of the bisphosphonates. *Bone*, *49*(1), 20-33.

112. Chavassieux, P. M., Arlot, M. E., Reda, C., Wei, L., Yates, A. J., & Meunier, P. J. (1997). Histomorphometric assessment of the long-term effects of Alendronate on bone quality and remodeling in patients with osteoporosis. *Journal of Clinical Investigation*, *100*(6), 1475.

113. Recker, R. R., Delmas, P. D., Halse, J., Reid, I. R., Boonen, S., García-Hernandez, P. A., & Hu, H. (2008). Effects of intravenous zoledronic acid once yearly on bone remodeling and bone structure. *Journal of Bone and Mineral Research*, *23*(1), 6-16.

114. Roschger, P., Rinnerthaler, S., Yates, J., Rodan, G. A., Fratzl, P., & Klaushofer, K. (2001). Alendronate increases degree and uniformity of mineralization in cancellous bone and decreases the porosity in cortical bone of osteoporotic women. *Bone*, *29*(2), 185-191.

115. Black, D. M., Cummings, S. R., Karpf, D. B., Cauley, J. A., Thompson, D. E., Nevitt, M. C., & Ott, S. M. (1996). Randomised trial of effect of Alendronate on risk of fracture in women with existing vertebral fractures. *The Lancet*, *348*(9041), 1535-1541.

116. Cummings, S. R., Black, D. M., Thompson, D. E., Applegate, W. B., Barrett-Connor, E., Musliner, T. A., & Vogt, T. (1998). Effect of Alendronate on risk of

fracture in women with low bone density but without vertebral fractures: results from the Fracture Intervention Trial. *Jama, 280*(24), 2077-2082.

117. Harris, S. T., Watts, N. B., Genant, H. K., McKeever, C. D., Hangartner, T., Keller, M., & Axelrod, D. W. (1999). Effects of Risedronate treatment on vertebral and nonvertebral fractures in women with postmenopausal osteoporosis: a randomized controlled trial. *Jama, 282*(14), 1344-1352.

118. Grbic, J. T., Landesberg, R., Lin, S. Q., Mesenbrink, P., Reid, I. R., Leung, P. C., & Eriksen, E. F. (2008). Incidence of osteonecrosis of the jaw in women with postmenopausal osteoporosis in the health outcomes and reduced incidence with zoledronic acid once yearly pivotal fracture trial. *The Journal of the American Dental Association, 139*(1), 32-40.

119. Shane, E., Burr, D., Ebeling, P. R., Abrahamsen, B., Adler, R. A., Brown, T. D., & Dempster, D. (2010). Atypical subtrochanteric and diaphyseal femoral fractures: report of a task force of the American Society for Bone and Mineral Research. *Journal of Bone and Mineral Research, 25*(11), 2267-2294.

120. Khosla, S., Burr, D., Cauley, J., Dempster, D. W., Ebeling, P. R., Felsenberg, D., & McCauley, L. K. (2007). Bisphosphonate-associated osteonecrosis of the jaw: report of a task force of the American Society for Bone and Mineral Research. *Journal of Bone and Mineral Research, 22*(10), 1479-1491.

121. Black, D. M., Schwartz, A. V., Ensrud, K. E., Cauley, J. A., Levis, S., Quandt, S. A., & Wehren, L. E. (2006). Effects of continuing or stopping Alendronate after 5 years of treatment: the Fracture Intervention Trial Long-term Extension (FLEX): a randomized trial. *Jama, 296*(24), 2927-2938.

122. Green, J., Czanner, G., Reeves, G., Watson, J., Wise, L., & Beral, V. (2010). Oral bisphosphonates and risk of cancer of oesophagus, stomach, and colorectum: case-control analysis within a UK primary care cohort. *Bmj, 341*, c4444.

123. Walker, A. M. (2014). Esophageal Cancer and Bisphosphonates. *Journal of Pharmaceutics & Drug Development, 2*(1), 1.

124. Adami, S., Bhalla, A. K., Dorizzi, R., Montesanti, F., Rosini, S., Salvagno, G., & Cascio, V. L. (1987). The acute-phase response after bisphosphonate administration. *Calcified tissue international, 41*(6), 326-331.

125. Rosen, C. J., & Brown, S. (2003). Severe hypocalcemia after intravenous bisphosphonate therapy in occult vitamin D deficiency. *New England Journal of Medicine, 348*(15), 1503-1504.

126. Beitz, J., Ibrahim, A., Scher, N., & Williams, G. (2003). Renal failure with the use of zoledronic acid. *N Engl J Med, 349*, 1676-1679.

127. Loke, Y. K., Jeevanantham, V., & Singh, S. (2009). Bisphosphonates and atrial fibrillation. *Drug safety, 32*(3), 219-228.

128. Watts, N. B., Chines, A., Olszynski, W. P., McKeever, C. D., McClung, M. R., Zhou, X., & Grauer, A. (2008). Fracture risk remains reduced one year after discontinuation of Risedronate. *Osteoporosis international, 19*(3), 365-372.

129. Black, D. M., Reid, I. R., Boonen, S., Bucci-Rechtweg, C., Cauley, J. A., Cosman, F., & Leung, P. C. (2012). The effect of 3 versus 6 years of Zoledronic acid treatment of osteoporosis: A randomized extension to the HORIZON-Pivotal Fracture Trial (PFT). *Journal of bone and mineral research, 27*(2), 243-254.

130. Kostenuik, P. J. (2005). Osteoprotegerin and RANKL regulate bone resorption, density, geometry and strength. *Current opinion in pharmacology*, *5*(6), 618-625.

131. Hu, M. I., Glezerman, I. G., Leboulleux, S., Insogna, K., Gucalp, R., Misiorowski, W., & Jaccard, A. (2014). Denosumab for treatment of hypercalcemia of malignancy. *The Journal of Clinical Endocrinology & Metabolism*, *99*(9), 3144-3152.

132. Torring, O. (2015). Effects of denosumab on bone density, mass and strength in women with postmenopausal osteoporosis. *Ther Adv Musculoskelet Dis*, 7(3), 88-102.

133. Block, G. A., Bone, H. G., Fang, L., Lee, E., & Padhi, D. (2012). A single-dose study of denosumab in patients with various degrees of renal impairment. *Journal of Bone and Mineral Research*, *27*(7), 1471-1479.

134. McClung MR, Lewiecki EM, Bolognese MA, *et al.* (2010) 233 8 year abstract. *ISCD* March.

135. Langdahl, B. L., Teglbjærg, C. S., Ho, P. R., Chapurlat, R., Czerwinski, E., Kendler, D. L., & Bolognese, M. A. (2015). A 24-month Study Evaluating the Efficacy and Safety of Denosumab for the Treatment of Men With Low Bone Mineral Density: Results From the ADAMO Trial. *The Journal of Clinical Endocrinology & Metabolism*.

136. Kong, Y. Y., Yoshida, H., Sarosi, I., Tan, H. L., Timms, E., Capparelli, C., & Khoo, W. (1999). OPGL is a key regulator of osteoclastogenesis, lymphocyte development and lymph-node organogenesis. *Nature*, *397*(6717), 315-323.

137. Bekker, P. J., Holloway, D. L., Rasmussen, A. S., Murphy, R., Martin, S. W., Leese, P. T., & DePaoli, A. M. (2004). A single-dose placebo-controlled study of AMG 162, a fully human monoclonal antibody to RANKL, in postmenopausal women. *Journal of Bone and Mineral Research*, *19*(7), 1059-1066.

138. Miller, P. D., Bolognese, M. A., Lewiecki, E. M., McClung, M. R., Ding, B., Austin, M., & San Martin, J. (2008). Effect of denosumab on bone density and turnover in postmenopausal women with low bone mass after long-term continued, discontinued, and restarting of therapy: a randomized blinded phase 2 clinical trial. *Bone*, *43*(2), 222-229.

139. Cheng, M. L., & Gupta, V. (2012). Teriparatide–indications beyond osteoporosis. *Indian journal of endocrinology and metabolism*, *16*(3), 343.

140. Brewer, H. B., Fairwell, T., Ronan, R., Sizemore, G. W., & Arnaud, C. D. (1972). Human parathyroid hormone: amino-acid sequence of the amino-terminal residues 1-34. *Proceedings of the National Academy of Sciences*, *69*(12), 3585-3588.

141. Dobnig, H., & Turner, R. T. (1995). Evidence that intermittent treatment with parathyroid hormone increases bone formation in adult rats by activation of bone lining cells. *Endocrinology*, *136*(8), 3632-3638.

142. Dobnig, H., & Turner, R. T. (1997). The Effects of Programmed Administration of Human Parathyroid Hormone Fragment (1–34) on Bone Histomorphometry and Serum Chemistry in Rats 1. *Endocrinology*, *138*(11), 4607-4612.

143. Lindsay, R., Nieves, J., Formica, C., Henneman, E., Woelfert, L., Shen, V., & Cosman, F. (1997). Randomised controlled study of effect of parathyroid hormone on vertebral-bone mass and fracture incidence among postmenopausal women on oestrogen with osteoporosis. *The Lancet, 350*(9077), 550-555.

144. Dobnig, H., Sipos, A., Jiang, Y., Fahrleitner-Pammer, A., Ste-Marie, L. G., Gallagher, J. C., Eriksen, E. F. (2005). Early changes in biochemical markers of bone formation correlate with improvements in bone structure during teriparatide therapy. *The Journal of Clinical Endocrinology & Metabolism, 90*(7), 3970-3977.

145. Neer, R. M., Arnaud, C. D., Zanchetta, J. R., Prince, R., Gaich, G. A., Reginster, J. Y., & Wang, O. (2001). Effect of parathyroid hormone (1-34) on fractures and bone mineral density in postmenopausal women with osteoporosis. *New England Journal of Medicine, 344*(19), 1434-1441.

146. Orwoll, E. S., Scheele, W. H., Paul, S., Adami, S., Syversen, U., Diez-Perez, A., & Gaich, G. A. (2003). The effect of teriparatide [human parathyroid hormone (1–34)] therapy on bone density in men with osteoporosis. *Journal of Bone and Mineral Research, 18*(1), 9-17.

147. Saag, K. G., Shane, E., Boonen, S., Marín, F., Donley, D. W., Taylor, K. A., & Marcus, R. (2007). Teriparatide or Alendronate in glucocorticoid-induced osteoporosis. *New England Journal of Medicine, 357*(20), 2028-2039.

148. Vahle, J. L., Long, G. G., Sandusky, G., Westmore, M., Ma, Y. L., & Sato, M. (2004). Bone neoplasms in F344 rats given teriparatide [rhPTH (1-34)] are dependent on duration of treatment and dose. *Toxicologic pathology, 32*(4), 426-438.

149. Prince, R., Sipos, A., Hossain, A., Syversen, U., Ish-Shalom, S., Marcinowska, E., & Mitlak, B. H. (2005). Sustained nonvertebral fragility fracture risk reduction after discontinuation of teriparatide treatment. *Journal of Bone and Mineral Research, 20*(9), 1507-1513.

150. Black, D. M., Bilezikian, J. P., Ensrud, K. E., Greenspan, S. L., Palermo, L., Hue, T., & Rosen, C. J. (2005). One year of Alendronate after one year of parathyroid hormone (1–84) for osteoporosis. *New England Journal of Medicine, 353*(6), 555-565.